BRITISH COLUMBIA CANCER AGENCY
LIBRARY
600 WEST 10th AVE.
VANCOUVER, B.C. CANADA
V5Z 4

D0575770

BRITISH COLUMBIA CANCER AGENCY
LIBRARY

BRITISH COLUMBIA CANCER AGENCY
LIBRARY
600 WEST 10th AVE.
VANCOUVER, B.C.   CANADA
V5Z 4E6

BRITISH COLUMBIA CANCER AGENCY
LIBRARY
600 WEST 10th AVE.
VANCOUVER, B.C.   CANADA
V5Z 4E6

COUNSELING PERSONS WITH CANCER

ABOUT THE AUTHOR

John V. Conti, Ph.D., C.R.C., N.C.C., has been a professional counselor for twenty years and a cancer survivor for eight years. He has been a volunteer for the American Cancer Society since 1982.

Dr. Conti is both a Certified Rehabilitation Counselor and a Nationally Certified Counselor. He is currently Assistant Regional Commissioner of the Rehabilitation Services Administration, United States Department of Education. The opinions expressed in this book are his own and do not necessarily represent the views of the Department of Education.

Dr. Conti, his wife of twenty-three years, Frances, and their two children, Matthew and Regina, live in New Hyde Park, New York.

COUNSELING PERSONS WITH CANCER

By

JOHN V. CONTI

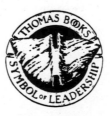

CHARLES C THOMAS • PUBLISHER
Springfield • Illinois • U.S.A.

Published and Distributed Throughout the World by

CHARLES C THOMAS • PUBLISHER
2600 South First Street
Springfield, Illinois 62794-9265

This book is protected by copyright. No part of
it may be reproduced in any manner without
written permission from the publisher.

© *1989 by* CHARLES C THOMAS • PUBLISHER

ISBN 0-398-05590-4

Library of Congress Catalog Card Number: 89-4436

With THOMAS BOOKS *careful attention is given to all details of manufacturing
and design. It is the Publisher's desire to present books that are satisfactory as to their
physical qualities and artistic possibilities and appropriate for their particular use.*
THOMAS BOOKS *will be true to those laws of quality that assure a good name
and good will.*

Printed in the United States of America
SC-R-3

Library of Congress Cataloging-in-Publication Data

Conti, John V.
    Counseling persons with cancer / by John V. Conti.
        p.   cm.
    Bibliography: p.
    Includes index.
    ISBN 0-398-05590-4
    1. Cancer—Patients—Counseling of.   2. Cancer.   I. Title.
RC262.C62   1989
616.99'4—dc 20   89-4436
                                                                  CIP

ACKNOWLEDGMENTS

This book is dedicated to the many persons who have endured cancer in their lives, and to their families and friends who have fought the disease, and lived the triumphs and disappointments along with them.

I am especially grateful to my wife Frances, and to my children, Matthew and Regina, for their love, patience, and understanding during the difficult days that became the impetus for the writing of this book. Their assistance and suggestions helped immeasurably.

The editorial skills of Eric Johnson benefited the manuscript tremendously and I am most grateful to him for being so generous with his time and talents.

CONTENTS

Contents

LIST OF CHARTS

COUNSELING PERSONS WITH CANCER

Chapter 1

INTRODUCTION

There is not much written information available for the counselor interested in counseling persons with cancer. With that lack in mind, a review of the most relevant materials is presented on the following pages, with a synthesis of current thinking offered. An overview of counseling theory and techniques is given, and a primer to understanding cancer follows. Causes and treatments are described in detail. Care was taken to present complex scientific concepts in a straightforward style, understandable to a layman. The writer combines the two specialized areas of counseling and cancer in the culminating section, which specifically focuses on counseling individuals with cancer, as well as their families. Special attention is devoted to a description of self-help methods. The author draws widely on his personal experience as a professional counselor, and as a person with a cancer history.

The central issue is that of support, particularly verbal support, for persons diagnosed as having cancer, as well as for their families. We will focus on the special nature of the relationship between the counselors and their clients, and the counseling knowledges and skills needed by the practitioner.

Counseling is defined as verbal intervention and ongoing interaction with one or more persons, and is used here to include the efforts of both lay and professional counselors. The terms "cancer patient" and "cancer client" are intended to encompass individuals who have been diagnosed as having any of the various forms of cancer and are receiving treatment, as well as persons who perceive themselves as high risk for cancer as a result of preliminary tests or symptoms. The fearfulness or "cancer phobia" of such persons often requires immediate and careful attention. A cancer patient or client also includes persons who have a previous history of the disease; sometimes they are referred to as "cancer survivors." Human service workers wonder what a non-medical practitioner needs to know about cancer in order to work effectively with cancer patients. How much understanding of the disease process is needed?

3

How much detail about the various forms of cancer is it necessary for the counselor to know? Many counselors lack specific knowledge about the onset of illness, prognosis, survival rates, and methods of medical intervention.

The differences between professional counseling and peer counseling will also be explored. What are the appropriate objectives and methods for both counselors? The ethical and realistic limitations of all forms of counseling, but especially of peer counseling, will be examined. The necessary background and preparation for various types of counseling is discussed, with specific distinctions among the following groups of practitioners as cancer counselors: physicians, including oncologists and psychiatrists; psychologists, social workers, and rehabilitation counselors; other mental health professionals, such as psychotherapists, nurses, clergymen, and family counselors; lay counselors with some limited training including cancer patients; and cancer survivors who have an interest in sharing their empathy, unique experiences, and insights.

Chapter 2

AN OVERVIEW OF THE COUNSELING TASK

Persons who experience life-threatening illness become changed individuals. Upon learning of a serious, and potentially life-threatening diagnosis, the most usual reaction is shock and confusion. It is critically important for these persons to receive clear and direct communication. This is called counseling. Information at this stage is usually conveyed by a physician, and it is rarely thought of as counseling by either the patient or the physician.

When the person who is ill needs to make decisions about accepting one or more forms of treatment, there is much need for information, but often little knowledge of where to obtain it. A helping person is needed to assist the diagnosed individual to understand, explore, and sort out the options available to him. When such a person is sought and found, and when this person participates in this process, he or she is a counselor, regardless of training, discipline, or professional credentials.

While the patient receives treatment, there is a continuing need to receive information, sort out feelings, and make plans for the future. These things are best accomplished within a counseling relationship.

Following active treatment, as patients begin to think of themselves as persons with a history of a life-threatening illness, or as survivors of that illness, they need counseling assistance to help them deal with the fear that the treatment was not effective or that the illness will recur, or to help them plan for their survivors if all treatments have been exhausted and they are deemed terminal. Even in cases where the fear of recurrence gradually recedes, as the patient survives in a healthy condition for an increasing length of time, patients/survivors often wish to take a new look at themselves, re-evaluate their philosophies of life, and change certain living habits which they feel may have contributed to their illness. Such people often seek help in finding answers to these questions or in examining possible future directions. The helper, in these cases, is a counselor.

5

Throughout the various stages of experiencing a life-threatening illness, and there are more stages than those briefly summarized above, there is always a need for an objective, caring person to assist the individual through the process. This is true without exception. Such a person is not always sought or accepted or found or up to the task. But he or she is always needed.

It does not have to be one person. It can be a series of people helping at various stages. They need not all be trained professionals. The acceptable backgrounds for such persons is broad and may range from sensitive lay persons to highly credentialed mental health professionals with specific training and experience in working with similar patients.

There are several illnesses that can be accurately described as life-threatening. As stated above, the illness that is focused on in this study is that of cancer. Readers familiar with other serious illnesses may find many similarities in the things observed about cancer patients and survivors and their own experiences with other illnesses. One would expect that some of the principles to be discussed, such as the emotional stages experienced by many cancer patients, are common to some people with other health problems. Many of the conclusions may be generalizable, as may some of the researcher's suggestions to patients and counselors. The principles and observations discussed, however, are made with the cancer patient in mind. The patients who were observed, relatives and friends who were interviewed, and the peer groups who were visited were all cancer related. No wider applications are claimed.

VERBAL SUPPORT: DISTINGUISHING AMONG FORMS OF SUPPORT

There are many forms of support that may be helpful to a person in a health crisis. Clearly, taking responsibility for tasks and errands, both related and unrelated to the health crisis, is an obvious example. "Can I do anything?" "Please let us know if there is any way we can help you." These are comments often heard by persons who have received the news that someone they know is suffering from cancer. They are frequently sincere in their offers of help, and people in trouble do accept, albeit selectively, assistance from those close to them.

A less tangible form of support is the sympathetic look, the pat on the arm, and the somber manner, posture, and body language that tells the person going through a health crisis that his plight is saddening and a source of concern to others. Some people reject this type of display and might argue that it is not even a form of support. Overdone (for example, a flood of tears accompanied by wailing) it can surely be offensive. But simple, sincere signs and murmurs of sympathy can be comforting to even the most sophisticated and unemotional of us when we are vulnerable, frightened, and in psychic pain.

COUNSELING DEFINED AND DELIMITED

Although doing practical tasks and offering sympathy and other signs of caring are bonafide forms of support, the form that will be dealt with primarily here is that of counseling. Counseling is usually a verbal ongoing interaction with one or more persons, and is used here to include the efforts of both lay counselors and professionally employed counselors. Most simply, to counsel is to give advice. But that description fails to provide an accurate picture of the process at its best. It is a form of intervention in which sensitive listening, timing, and the highest respect for feelings are of critical importance. Counseling may be more fully defined as verbal intervention aimed at allowing an individual in distress, or otherwise in need of advice or direction, to see his situation more clearly and objectively and to gain the understanding needed to arrive at a solution. The latter may result in accepting the situation, as unpleasant as it may be, or in trying to change things, relying on newly found understandings and insights. The counselor must carefully listen and try to understand everything the client says, everything he doesn't say, and form some appreciation of the content and the tone of the remarks. The experienced counselor does not hastily interpret the client's remarks, nor hurry to share premature analysis or interpretations with the client. He reflects feelings and asks questions so he can understand the client. He explores why the client discusses one area and not another. He appreciates the client's vulnerability and he understands that clients often develop a close bond with the counselor. In psychotherapy this continuing, intense closeness and affection is referred to as **transference** and is often traced to feelings the client has had with other persons in his life. In cancer counseling, transference does not occur as readily as in psychoanalytic counseling because cancer counseling is often short term, issue-based, and dominated by health concerns. The counselor working with cancer patients often finds himself being much more directive—actively guiding, advising, directing the discussion—than when working with other clients. This is brought about by the many decisions that need to be resolved quickly. Non-directive counseling can be more effectively employed when the client's concerns are more general; for example, anxiety feelings, lack of confidence in one's abilities, and problems of self-acceptance or self-esteem. In this situation, the counselor speaks much less, concentrates on reflecting feelings, displays an unconditional positive regard toward the client, and gently guides the client toward a better self-awareness and acceptance as well as a clearer understanding of needs, motivations, behaviors, and appreciation of his uniqueness and strengths.

A PATIENT IS A CLIENT IS A COUNSELEE

The reader may have noticed that in the above discussion, the person with cancer suddenly became a "client." An individual receiving counseling is referred to in many ways, depending often on the orientation, training, and professional discipline of the counselor, as well as the setting in which the counseling takes place. Physicians advise their "patients." Psychotherapists also refer to the people they counsel as "patients." In peer counseling, the lay counselor sometimes thinks of both himself and his counselee as "patients," especially if medical treatment is still being administered. Nurses and other medically oriented personnel, some of whom have developed counseling practices, almost always use the term "patient."

Most rehabilitation counselors, guidance counselors, career and employment counselors, family and marriage counselors, and vocational counselors speak of their "clients." The setting of employment often determines which term—patient or client—is used. If a social worker is employed in a vocationally oriented rehabilitation agency, he is taught to think in terms of "clients," but if he works in a community mental health agency, he probably speaks of his "patients."

Since the author's training and background are in both rehabilitation counseling and psychology, the individual receiving counseling is sometimes referred to as a "client," especially in the section about rehabilitation. But the term "patient" is also used, especially in those places where the term seems to convey a more accurate description of what the person is probably feeling and experiencing.

WORKING WITH THOSE PERSONS
CLOSE TO THE CLIENT

Counseling persons dealing with a cancer diagnosis often necessitates the need for working with other people in the client's life. This is most often the client's spouse, child, or parent, but could also be an unmarried life partner, a companion or a close friend. Many times "significant others" feel a degree of shock and trauma that rivals the intensity of the client's.

In some cases, the counselor meets a family member or a friend at the outset since that individual was responsible for referring the client. Unfortunately this type of referral is not the most promising. Self-referral is best in terms of the client accepting the need for counseling assistance, but referral from another professional worker is almost as good. When family members or friends of a newly diagnosed patient initiate the counseling intervention, often the patient will resist. Risk of failure is even greater when the well-meaning relative or friend speaks first with the counselor in an attempt to "pave the way." Fortunately, most cancer patients are not coerced into seeing a counselor. When the counselor meets an important person in the client's life through the client's suggestion or request, an initial rapport is established. This rapport should not damage the relationship between the counselor and the client.

Some clients feel more comfortable when accompanied by a relative or a friend for the first interview. This should be allowed. If possible, however, the counselor should attempt to see the client alone for at least part of the time, whether by calling in the client first (assuring that the friend or relative will soon be asked to join the session), or by allowing a little time alone with the client at the end of the session. This may be done casually by saying something like: "Fred, I wonder if you would mind if Sylvia and I spent a few minutes alone. We sometimes find that it helps us to get to know each other a little better and helps to get things started off well. If you would wait in the other room, I promise to send her right out to you." Friends and relatives rarely, if ever, protest. If the client is very apprehensive or the companion very protective the counselor should not insist upon seeing them separately. This might be attempted at the following session.

Most clients, but especially persons with cancer, need the option of speaking one-on-one with a counselor. Too often, cancer patients in conjoint sessions will withhold fears and feelings in a misguided concern for those close to them. Eventually, the counselor may determine that this is not the case, and that in fact participating in counseling together would be the most beneficial course of action. An example of such a situation is when a woman has had a mastectomy and is concerned about her husband's feelings. Seeing a counselor together allows some couples to relate more easily to each other in sharing some difficult, sensitive, and painful feelings. Even in this case, however, it is usually best for the woman to meet with a counselor alone for a period of time before beginning conjoint sessions. It is important for her to express her shock, anger, fear, and disappointment, as well as her hopes for the future, before becoming overly involved with the perceptions and feelings of those around her.

Occasionally the counselor runs into a situation where it is apparent that the family member or the friend needs individual counseling. This person's problem may be related to the client's cancer diagnosis, or it may be totally unrelated. Before the counselor decides to take on the companion as an additional client, he must predict the effect of doing so. The counselor may decide the companion requires some individual counseling. If that is the case, the counselor should refer him or her to another counselor. If he decides to see both individually, he will need to assure them that their sessions are confidential. This can usually be accomplished simply by the counselor's manner and by what he does not say, rather than by making promises in advance or chastizing the client if he asks about what was revealed in the other's session. If the client hints for such revelations the counselor can gently tell him that it is important that all clients enjoy the comfort and freedom of speaking without fear of what they say being shared with others.

The counselor's relationship with persons close to his client may, therefore, be non-existent, it may be restricted to a casual telephone conversation or it can develop into a counselor-client relationship. Rarely is family therapy needed as a direct result of a cancer experience. When therapy is indicated for a family of three or more it is usually because the family has been having other problems and the cancer experience triggered a crisis. When this occurs, the counselor should evaluate his own comfort and confidence in working with the family. If he has questions about his competence, he must either seek assistance from a more experienced counselor or refer his client to a worker trained in family therapy.

Chapter 3

CRUCIAL COMPONENTS
OF COUNSELING PRACTICE

THEORIES, GOALS, TECHNIQUES

As we mentioned earlier, many professional persons strive to bring about constructive change of attitude in their clients through multiple face-to-face contacts. Regardless of what he calls himself, he is essentially engaged in counseling, and hopefully some of his clients emerge from the process somewhat better adjusted to their problems.

Assisting persons in difficulty may be attempted by manipulating the environment (such as removing a child from his home and placing him in a foster home or transferring a worker from one department to another) or by employing techniques to help a maladjusted individual gain a better understanding of his situation. Counseling and psychotherapy fall into this latter category. These two approaches are not the only means of assisting individuals. Other adjustment techniques include the various so-called "expressive therapies," such as psychodrama, play therapy, and art therapy. Even dietary, hormonal treatments, and surgical interventions may be considered means of altering behavior (Rogers, 1942). We will limit further discussion of readjustment techniques to counseling, although it is clearly not the only avenue for improving one's outlook on life.

In the view of some, the single purpose of counseling is to facilitate development (Tyler, 1961). There are many counseling orientations and philosophies. A type of counseling called "developmental counseling," promoted by Blocher, has a primary goal of maximizing human freedom and effectiveness. He sees counseling and psychotherapy primarily aimed at changing human behavior. There are two described outcomes of counseling and psychotherapy in Blocher's system—the first is developmental-educative-preventive; the second is a cluster of remediative-adjustive-therapeutic outcomes. He sees developmental counseling as being concerned with the first group. The second set of

11

goals or outcomes are related to adjustment to certain situations, resolving conflicts, and breaking down and replacing defenses. Blocher makes elaborate distinctions between counseling and psychotherapy. Some of his major points of distinction are that (1) clients who come for counseling are not considered mentally ill, (2) counseling is focused on the present and future—not the past, (3) the counselor is not an authority figure who creates an illusion of omnipotence through a transference relationship, (4) counselors do not attempt to hide their own feelings, values, and standards from their clients, and (5) the counselor focuses on changing behavior—not creating insight. Blocher asserts that therapists do not actually change the "constructs" that have been used to describe or explain behavior; for example, concepts such as ego strength and personality core. He believes that the only useful process is one that emphasizes changing human behavior and facilitating development through a direct educational approach (Blocher, 1966).

A psychoanalytic approach to counseling is espoused by Bordin, who defines the psychological counselor as someone who assists people with problems, often behavioral problems, in which the critical issues are most often related to motivations and emotions. People are seen as wanting to reduce tensions. The individual learns at a very young age that unbridled expression of urges is punished. These impulses, therefore, become modified in the form of various defenses against anxiety. Human motivation is largely seen as unconscious (Bordin, 1955).

The orthodox analytic view, as explained by Freud and others, is that, in the therapeutic process, the patient gives up his efforts to keep his impulses from awareness and starts reacting to situations and people in terms of their **present** demands, rather than as though they were repeating demands made in childhood. Surrendering the defenses can only be done in a transference situation. In this way, the unconscious can be made conscious. The patient's unconsummated impulses, both aggressive and loving, will center on the therapist. The psychoanalytic counselor interprets by calling attention to unconscious aspects of the patient's behavior and points out when he is resisting. Although resistance reduces anxiety, it blocks forward movement in the analysis. Counseling does not try to bring infantile conflicts to the surface and resolve them, although ways in which these conflicts appear in conscious acions may be examined.

Rogers borrowed much from the Freudians in developing his nondirective, client-centered, counseling theory. His central theme is the person's need for self-enhancement. Like the Freudians, he stresses the importance of experiences that have been denied awareness. Maladjustment, to Rogers, is the result of experiences becoming assimilated in distorted form into self-perception. The more experience that is denied to awareness, the greater difficulty in maintaining a consistent self-concept. The result may be that eventually neurotic systems may develop as ways of satisfying needs which must be denied to awareness in order to maintain "self-consistency."

Non-directive therapeutic thought sees resistance as the result of misdirected therapeutic effort and not as the psychoanalytic view would assert, as an inevitable part of the therapeutic process. The therapist can avoid resistance in the client by avoiding guiding and evaluating behaviors and therefore can concentrate on accepting the client. Also unlike the psychoanalysts, Rogers states that transference is not necessary for therapeutic progress. It is necessary, however, that the therapist step into the client's frame of reference and understand his world as he sees it (Rogers, 1942).

Rank, Taft, Allen, and Borden were all influenced by Rogerian thinking and developed psychological counseling theories of their own which are derivative, but depart from Rogers in varied ways. Bordin, for example, believes that resistance is an important aspect of the therapeutic relationship. He agrees with Rogers that resistance may result from the client's reaction to an inappropriate interpretation or a lack of acceptance by the therapist, but he sides with the psychoanalysts in saying that resistance basically arises from internally determined anxiety. Bordin states that transference is a crucial part of psychotherapy but, leaning toward the non-directive view, believes it is possible to overcome repression without the presence of transference.

The many counseling theorists disagree on various points, even when they are in basic agreement in a counseling approach. In terms of diagnosis, Rogers is strongly opposed to using diagnostic labels because he sees it as evaluating the client, and therefore threatening, making a permissive atmosphere impossible. Psychoanalysis stresses the importance of interpretation as a form of rejection. Allen also minimizes interpretations. Fenichel says that the major goal of therapy is simply for the client to become aware of his feelings. Nearly everyone agrees that counseling is likely to be more cognitive than therapy (Bordin, 1955).

It has been said that understanding the client fosters a feeling of security **in the counselor.** Counselors do different things at different times with different clients. Each of these things is intended to be therapeutic or problem-solving in some way. Counselors choose to employ varied therapeutic techniques because of differential understandings. If the counselor's understandings are of the moment-to-moment feelings of the client, he is apt to use techniques such as reflection, clarification, and simple acceptance of feelings. But if the counselor is operating in terms of personality structure concepts, then he is more likely to use the techniques of interpretation and information-giving (Callis, Polmantier, Roeber, 1955).

Some counselors become confused with the myriad theories of human behavior and proper counselor technique that are promoted in the literature. It is comforting to remember that studies have demonstrated that expert psychotherapists create better relationships with clients than novices. Hence experience alone will lead to improvement, regardless of philosophical orientation. Moreover, the therapeutic relationship created by experts of one school resembles the relationship created by experts of other schools more closely than it does the relationship created by non-experts of the same school. Finally, the most important dimension differentiating experts from non-experts is related to the therapist's ability to understand the patient and to communicate and maintain rapport with him (Fiedler, 1950 (2)).

Directive counseling techniques include developing the problem for the client. The counselor takes the initiative by searching different areas of client behavior and thought in order to develop the problem. "How would you describe your family?" and "What sort of grades are you getting?" are examples of this type of direct investigation.

The non-directive counselor takes less initiative. He will reflect the client's statements and clarify to the point where the client takes the lead in developing the problem. Rogers espoused a mild form of interpretation which he called clarification. The counselor may assist the client in reaching self-understanding by reformulating insights which have already been arrived at and accepted.

The most non-directive therapist must keep some control over the interview, even if it is simply to set limits within which the counseling occurs.

McGowan's very straightforward advice is to avoid being authoritative, be frank but sensitive, get the facts, and don't ask "yes" and "no" questions. Other suggestions are to communicate warmth, understanding, and acceptance, and avoid evaluating and overidentifing with the client (McGowan, 1960).

Snyder examined psychological counseling in an attempt to measure the frequency of various psychotherapeutic methods. He found that clarification of feeling comprises about half of counselors' statements. Counselors made structuring, persuasive, critical, and disapproving comments less than 10 percent of the time. Simple acceptance accounted for 25 percent of the counselor's remarks. In examining client statements, it is interesting that one third of the client's remarks were classified as statement of his problem, while 12 percent were indicative of understanding and insight (Brayfield, 1950). Client talk also was examined by Carnes and Robinson, who concluded that the amount of client talk yielded a low positive correlation with insight and the extent of the working relationship between client and counselor, and a high positive correlation with the degree of client responsibility for the progress of the session. As one would guess, clients working with non-directive counselors spoke more than clients whose counselors were classified as directive, but the former clients showed no greater degree of insight than the latter. The authors concluded that the amount of client talk could not be used as a criteria for determining the effectiveness of the counseling (Brayfield, 1950).

Patterson warns counselors against "doing things" for clients. It is important to counsel toward client independence. The counselor must resist helping the client with specific problems the client can solve for himself, even when it would be easier for the counselor to do so (Patterson, 1960).

In discussing various counseling theories, some exploration of techniques was mentioned in illustrating principal concepts. Some further discussion of technique might be useful in examining what actually occurs in a counseling relationship.

In counseling situations of a non-directive character, insight (defined as new understandings and perceptions of the self) develops in a spontaneous manner, according to Rogers. It follows free expression of negative emotion, and is likely to develop if the counselor uses responses which are clarifying and accepting. Procedures which make the client feel completely understood, while not causing defensiveness, are reported to be the most successful (Brayfield, 1950).

Some counselors point out that the counseling relationship itself is a "counseling method." This view is in agreement with those who regard transference as a critical component of the counseling process. Transference is a very central concept in psychological counseling or therapy. A phenomenon of interpersonal relationships, transference is best seen, recognized, and studied in psychoanalysis. According to Thompson, transference consists of irrational attitudes toward another person, usually an authority figure. He believes that it can be used as a therapeutic instrument in all forms of psychotherapy. Counselors study the irrational trends and investigate their origins, and try to determine what the patient is attempting to achieve. This should lead to a modification and disappearance of the irrational thinking, through **insight**. Although the process described is the ideal in psychoanalytic work, an alternate approach is to use the extreme degree of authority which the patient has endowed the therapist with, to **influence** the patient. With this approach, there is no effort toward destroying the irrational overevaluation of the therapist, but rather utilizing it to give power to positive advice and recommendations. The approach is risky, however, since the patient may become hostile or develop a prolonged dependency. The patient presumably does not understand his feelings as this process is ongoing. Some therapists cite time factors as a reason for utilizing a therapeutic approach. If you hope to achieve a quick cure, you may not be able to take the time for the patient to develop insight. This leads some therapists to more controversial methods, such as narcoanalysis and hypnoanalysis, to rapidly decrease negative symptoms (Brayfield, 1950).

Patients who are hospitalized are particularly prone to transference. Professionals in the hospital apparently remind patients of earlier ministering figures (Patterson, 1960).

Thorne agrees with those who see the process as primarily educational. This philosophy directs the counselor to make available a wide variety of resources, allowing the client to learn more adequate ways of solving his problems. He speaks of his approach as "directive psychotherapy" (Brayfield, 1950).

Lofquist advocates behavior midway between directive and nondirective. There should be a genuine interaction with neither the counselor nor the client becoming prominent in the communication. The counselor should be active — not passive — and should facilitate the client's learning by structuring the learning situation (Patterson, 1960).

Counseling is not something you **do**, but rather something you engage in **with** a client. It is, therefore, most importantly a **relationship**. The principles are those that foster good mental health; self-esteem, which the counselor can promote through acceptance and respect; understanding;

confidence; and trust. All good human relationships are also character-ized by honesty, integrity, and openness. If the counselor follows these principles, the client will move forward. If threat is present, however, learning will not occur (Patterson, 1960).

The counselor is elsewhere described as a collaborator. He collabo-rates with a counselee in a process devoted to exploring one's self, gaining new perceptions, and solving problems. This occurs in a psycho-logical climate which is both intimate and objective. The client has complete freedom in expressing his point of view; that is what makes the process intimate. But since the viewpoint is examined and clarified, it is also objective (Buchheimer and Balogh, 1961). The counselee is seen here as a person on a quest. His quest stems from dissatisfaction with some aspect of himself, or the dissatisfaction of others with him, or, less frequently, with his dissatisfaction with others.

Acquiring counseling skills and techniques can only be partially taught. The techniques discussed need ultimately to be integrated into the individual's personal counseling style (Buchheimer and Balogh, 1961).

Fiedler's research indicated that the crucial factor in the success of counseling or therapy is the counselor's ability to communicate his understanding of the client's point of view (Fieldler, 1950 (1) (2)).

In discussing roles of the rehabilitation counselor, Anderson points out that what all definitions have in common is that the counselor concerns himself with the motivations and attitudes of his client. There is an assumption that clients have adjustment problems which will be the focus of the counseling process. Above all, the counselor must be able to create a situation conducive to the client expressing his full attitudinal-motivational structure, and he must be skilled in creating a warm thera-peutic climate (Patterson, 1960).

A chart in the book entitled *The Counseling Relationship* lists a num-ber of techniques that a counselor may use. These techniques are meant to elicit feeling. The counselor's roles when using these techniques include receiving, accepting, and understanding. Techniques that are designed to facilitate self-understanding are tentative analysis, summari-zation, direct question, general leads, reassurance, and information giving. The respective counselor roles for those techniques are understanding, investigating, searching, explaining, supporting, and predicting. Listed techniques to bring about counselee action are encouragement, specific suggestion, urging and cajoling (!). These correspond to the counselor roles of predicting, advising, and directing. The authors provide sample types of communications to illustrate each (Buchheimer and Balogh, 1961).

As Carl Rogers refined his theory of client-centered counseling, he developed nineteen propositions on which his approach is based. A number of implications for counseling are derived from his theoretical framework. One is that the counselee is the best source of information about himself. So called objective or external measures are of little value. Establishing a relationship is the counselor's prime goal. Developing the relationship follows not from a set of techniques, but as a result of proper attitudes on the counselor's part. The counselor must experience genuine feelings of **unconditional positive regard** for the client or the relationship will not develop properly. Also, the counselor needs to be genuinely empathetic and understanding of the client, or, as Rogers refers to it, of the client's **internal frame of reference.** The major job of the counselor is to facilitate the client's own self-exploration through reflecting and clarifying feelings. Long periods of silence may be helpful in allowing the counselee to think through his situation. Rogers does not encourage counselors to provide information or assist in solving immediate problems. Treatment is similar for all cases. There is no distinction made between counseling and psychotherapy. Rogers promotes good training for counselors, but emphasizes that the most essential thing is for the counselor to have (1) his own profitable therapeutic experience that allows him to develop personal maturity and (2) the security that enables him to help others (Blocher, 1966; Rogers, 1951).

In counseling there is also an approach based on a social-psychological model. It stems from the psychoanalytic movement, but became modified by practitioners such as Sullivan, Adler, Fromm, and Horney. This group all modified Freud's thinking by making the assumption that personality develops as a result of social learning. Concepts such as **style of life** and **interpersonal strategies** as well as other forms of social interaction are critical to these theorists.

Albert Ellis promotes a **rational-emotive** therapy which operates on the assumption that emotions are controlled by easily understood cognitive, ideational processes. Emotions can be examined, changed, and rebuilt. Unhappiness comes from the way we react to the world's trials—not from the circumstances themselves. The counselor who follows Ellis's philosophy attempts to determine what false beliefs on which the client is basing irrational responses. He then points out the irrational elements while encouraging the client to try new alternative behaviors (Ellis, 1962; Blocher, 1966).

Behavioral counselors listen carefully to what responses increase the probability of recurrence of the response. These are called **reinforcers.** B.F. Skinner first pointed out that the study of stimuli and responses under controlled conditions can lead to modifying behavior by manipulating the situation through the use of reinforcers. In the counseling setting, it has been shown by many workers that behavior can be changed by manipulating verbal reinforcers. Operant conditioning and other implications of the behavioral approach have been used lately to extinguish unwanted behaviors, such as overeating, smoking, or phobic disorders.

Donald Crawford has done considerable work at the University of Buffalo in developing a comprehensive list of skills pertinent to rehabilitation counselors. He used items from the works of Matkin, Muthard, Salomone, Rubin, et al. and others, and came up with an inventory that is quite exhaustive. It includes employment development, placement counseling and follow-up, job analysis and modification, service planning, monitoring progress, consultation with other agencies and professionals, professional development, case recording and documentation, test administration development and interpretation, vocational counseling supervision, psychological theory and technique, as well as a separate category called special problems. The latter includes items such as "assesses suicide risk of clients," "possesses knowledge about acquired immune deficiency syndrome (AIDS) and works effectively with clients diagnosed with this illness," and "counsels traumatic brain injury clients." Of particular interest in Crawford's taxonomy is his listing of "Counseling Skills and Processes." This area includes 44 items and is reproduced here in its entirety since it allows us to synthesize the various theories, approaches, counseling concepts, and techniques that have been discussed in the above sections. The reader will note that items draw from the various schools of counseling thought and include very broad issues, such as "adjusts counseling approaches or styles according to client cognitive and personality characteristics," as well as extremely narrow, practical items, such as "reviews instructions with naive, retarded, or immature clients to be sure they use prescribed medication properly."

CHART 1

Counseling Skills and Processes

1. Provides facilitative conditions of empathy, respect and genuineness.
2. Promotes the establishment of rapport and self-exploration.
3. Uses awareness of personal impact to enhance counselor-client relationship and contribute to counseling goals.
4. Addresses relevant issues when counseling the racially or culturally different client, i.e., knows how to facilitate rapport and overcome barriers.
5. Requests supervision when strong personal reactions are elicited by certain clients.
6. Identifies one's own biases and weaknesses which may affect the development of a healthy client relationship.
7. Adjusts counseling approaches or styles according to client cognitive and personality characteristics.
8. Interprets diagnostic information to clients in a clear and tactful (considered) manner.
9. Assists clients in terminating counseling in a positive manner, thus enhancing their ability to function independently.
10. Recognizes serious psychological problems requiring immediate intervention through consultation, referral, or hospitalization (e.g., severe depression, suicidal ideation).
11. Explores client's needs for individual, group, or family counseling.
12. Counsels clients to help them appreciate and emphasize their personal assets.
13. Identifies alternative coping mechanisms that client may have to adjust to a problem.
14. Reflects feeling tone the client expresses to help him clarify his problems.
15. Appraises the extent and quality of the client's interpersonal relationships.
16. Discusses the client's interpersonal relationships in order to help him/her better understand their nature and quality.
17. Identifies alternative coping mechanisms that clients may have to adjust to a problem.
18. Talks with the client's relatives concerning problems arising from rehabilitation services, training, etc.
19. Evaluates the family's interest, involvement, and cooperation in the rehabilitation process.
20. Counsels with a client's family to provide information and support positive coping behaviors.
21. Reduces the client's anxiety by helping him/her face and realistically assess problems that seem insurmountable.
22. Interprets the motivations underlying clients behavior in order to identify relevant issues and aid in modifying clients' behavior.
23. Confronts clients with observations about inconsistencies between their goals and their behavior.
24. Recognizes and deals with transference and resistance as they arise during the client's psychotherapy to help him perceive the neurotic nature of his interpersonal relationships.
25. Counsels clients to help them understand or change their feelings about themselves and others.
26. Reflects feeling tone the client expresses to help him clarify his problems.
27. Helps clients work through dependency issues.
28. Evaluates the degree of client participation in the rehabilitation process.
29. Clarifies for clients mutual expectations and the nature of the counseling relationship.
30. Assists clients in verbalizing specific behavioral goals for personal adjustment.

31. Works with clients to identify mutually acceptable methods to resolve conflicts.
32. Uses assessment information to provide clients with insights into personal dynamics, e.g. denial or distortion.
33. Assists clients in modifying their lifestyles to accommodate functional limitations.
34. Assists clients in understanding stress and utilizing mechanisms for coping.
35. Counsels client regarding sexual concerns related to the presence of a disability.
36. Counsels the client to help him/her achieve an emotional and intellectual acceptance of the limitations imposed by the disability.
37. Helps clients develop responses to others' questions and comments about their disabilities.
38. Examines with clients the consequences of their disability and its significance in relation to work, family, and self-sufficiency.
39. Communicates with clients' relatives concerning adjustment to the disability.
40. Uses counseling methods to help the unemployable client accept and adjust to his unemployability.
41. Discusses the client's personal hygiene habits with him.
42. Conducts intake or screening interviews or both to determine how the counselor and his agency can help the client.
43. Reviews instructions with naive, retarded, or immature clients to be sure they use prescribed medication properly.
44. Helps clients, through group procedures, to learn and use new ways to deal with their problems.

(Crawford, 1987)

Chapter 4

CANCER

DEFINITION

Cancer is a disease, or more correctly a group of diseases, character-ized by abnormal cell growth. The uncontrollable and disordered growth of these cells can spread, and, if not stopped, will result in death.

Cancer has been regarded with dread and hopelessness by people for centuries. It was feared even by ancient civilizations by people whose lives were filled with uncertainty and threats to survival. The ancient Greeks gave cancer its name, which means "the crab." It was, throughout history, regarded as a death sentence. Only within the past twenty years have the fatal image and hopeless fear begun to fade (Clark et al., 1985; Renneker & Leib, 1979).

HISTORY

In their book, *Understanding Cancer,* Mark Renneker and Steven Leib report that the earliest known cancer was a blood vessel tumor of a vertebra reported in the fossil of a dinosaur from the Mesozoic era (125 million B.C.). In 1891 bone remains were unearthed which showed traces of cancer in a Java man (1 million B.C.). Ancient Egyptian writings refer to tumors and to primitive attempts to remove them by knife. Bone cancer was identified in mummies in the Great Pyramid of Gizeh (2500–1500 B.C.). Hypocrites recognized and described cancer of the breast, uterus, stomach, skin, and rectum. He coined the term **carcinoma** to refer to spreading tumors, as distinct from **benign tumors.** He burned away tissues with a hot iron as a treatment (cautery) and used caustic pastes (400 B.C.). Celsus, a Roman physician, performed the first human cancer surgery. Many mastectomies were later performed by other Roman physicians, without the benefit of anesthesia (100 A.D.).

According to Renneker and Leib, during the eighteenth century per-sons with cancer were thought to be highly contagious and they were

23

treated like lepers. Henri Ledran determined that cancer may spread through lymphatic channels to other sites in the body, and therefore promoted surgery as the only effective treatment. Sir Percival Pott published an early case of occupational-environmental cancer in chimney sweeps. In England, unclothed children were forced to climb narrow chimneys to clean the soot. When they became adults many of these chimney sweeps developed scrotal cancer as a result of the irritation caused by prolonged contact with soot (1775). Like Sir Percival, Richard von Volkmann described an early case of occupational-environmental cancer. Von Volkmann described how tar workers in Germany often developed cancer on their arms and hands from prolonged contact with tar.

Although tuberculosis was the leading cause of death in the United States in the nineteenth century, cancer claimed a great many lives. Stomach cancer was the most common form of cancer. Twice as many women as men died from cancer. During this period the average life expectancy was 40 years (1876).

Understanding Cancer reports that the first U.S. cancer hospital was established in New York City in 1884. Called Memorial Sloan-Kettering, today this hospital remains a major cancer treatment center. The radical mastectomy was first demonstrated in 1894 at The Johns Hopkins School of Medicine by William Halstead. His method is still the primary one in use today. Wilhelm Röntgen discovered a "penetrating ray," and in 1898 Pierre and Marie Curie opened the way for radiology with their isolation of radium. Many early radiologists later died of radiation-induced tumors. The American Cancer Society was founded in 1913. Sidney Farber successfully tested a new synthetic drug on children with leukemia in Boston. This 1947 development marked the beginnings of chemotherapy (Renneker & Leib, 1979).

DEVELOPMENT OF CANCER—THE PROCESS

Cancer can attack any of the body's organs. There are more than 250 different types of cancer and they all have one thing in common—they are the result of abnormal cell growth. Cells in all mammals divide and in so doing go through what is called a cell cycle.

The process is explained in the booklet called *Cancer Treatment* in the U.S. Department of Health and Human Service's *Medicine for the Layman* series. We don't fully understand how cancer develops, but we do know that the cell receives a signal that causes it to divide. When the cell starts to divide it doubles the amount of genetic materials—called *DNA*—in the nucleus of the cell. After the cell divides, there is a time of rest, followed by a breaking apart of the genetic material. This is called **mitosis.** The deoxyribonucleic acid (DNA) separates into two separate poles and then becomes two distinct cells. After mitosis the process may be repeated, or there may be a prolonged period of rest.

In observing 100 cancer cells, 10 to 20 of them will be seen continuously dividing, piling up many new cancer cells. The body contains different types of tissue: **static, expanding,** and **renewing.** Static tissue loses its capacity to divide when it reaches normal adult size. Muscle and nerve cells fall into this category. Unfortunately, when these types of cells are lost they cannot be replaced. Expanding tissue stops growing when it reaches normal adult size, but it can divide genetic material in its cells and replace cells that are removed. Although normally at rest, expanding tissue has the capacity to switch on if needed. For example, if half of a liver or a kidney is removed, the organ will expand to its normal size, and then stop.

Renewing tissue renews cells daily. However, adult renewing cells have a finite life span. The skin, intestinal tract lining, blood cells, and sperm cells are examples of renewing cells. Since white blood cells live less than a week, they require constant replacement. If some superficial skin is scraped off a finger, the body will recognize that cells have been lost, and the layer of skin responsible for replenishing cells will switch on and make new skin cells. Renewing cells are similar to cancer cells in the way they continually divide and grow. For this reason there are often problems with this type of cell when cancer is being treated with drugs. Normal tissues composed of renewing cells are vulnerable to change; these changes are called **side effects** (U.S. Dept. of H.H.S., 1984).

Unlike normal cells that grow to an appropriate number and then stop—having reached, for instance, the needed size for a liver or the required number of white blood cells in the bloodstream—cancer cells continue to grow crazily. Regardless of the size of mass it is producing, the cells continue to divide. Although it is not known why this happens, it is clearly related to the signal that stimulates the cell to divide. The cell may receive a signal it no longer understands, or it may not receive the normal signal to stop growing, or it may receive no signal (U.S. Dept. of H.H.S., 1984).

The greatest danger of cancer is that it invades and destroys normal tissue. Early in the process, cancer cells are confined to an original site, and the disease is said to be **localized.** But later some of the cells may move into neighboring tissue or organs, or they may travel to distant parts of the body (American Cancer Society, 1980).

Cancer cells can enter the blood stream and the lymphatic system, which drains the tissues, and thereby spreads the cancer cells around the body. This process is called **metastasis.** If the spread is confined to one region of the body, trapped by lymph nodes, it is termed **regional.** Without effective treatment the cancer will continue to spread, and lead to **advanced cancer,** usually culminating in death.

Secondary tumors can grow in parts of the body distant from the original site. A kidney cancer may have a metastatic tumor growing in the lungs and one in the brain. This leads to crowding of normal organs, a condition that will be fatal. In an enclosed area such as the brain, the cells expand to a point where they actually crush the organ making it no longer able to function. Another development leading to death is when the cancer cells use up the food supply available to the patient. Researchers have studied the progression of cancer in many individuals, and it is now known where the likely secondary sites will be for a metastatic colony to develop, based on the original site. This permits physicians and patients to be alert for signs and symptoms in these high risk areas.

In very early or embryonic, stages of normal development, cells grow at a rapid rate, similar to the rate at which cancer cells grow. As adulthood is reached, the growth rate has slowed down to a steady rate which insures that the number of new cells made equals the number of old cells lost. Cancer cells do not slow down until the end stage when the cells have run out of food and the blood supply shuts down, causing the patient to die.

When a cancer first develops it immediately begins to shed some of its cells through the lymphatics and blood stream. When scientists discovered this in the mid 1950s it was puzzling because it raised the question of how any cancer patient could survive. If all cancers shed cells, and if these cells are carried to distant parts of the body, then surgically removing the original growth should not, logically speaking, do away with the cancer since presumably cancer cells circulating throughout the body could take hold elsewhere. But about 20 years ago it was learned that the human **immune system** can kill cancer cells circulating in the blood. Patients therefore may not die when the original tumor begins shedding cancer cells.

The immune system is composed of **lymphocytes.** After receiving a defensive signal, lymphocytes called **B cells** and **T cells** form and protect the body. The thymus gland is one origin of this defensive signal. Researchers continue to search for a second organ believed to play a role in signaling the development of these protective cells. Antibodies that are produced by B cells fight infection; they also fight cancer. Together with a different cell, called a **macrophage,** T cell variants are known to directly attack cancer. A great deal about this whole process is still unknown. But it appears that the cancer cell membrane undergoes certain changes which are recognized by the immune cell. The characteristics of the membrane are thought to be unique to the virus or chemical agent that caused the malignancy. Thus, some cancer cells can be killed by the natural host immunity. But unfortunately the immune system can only deal with a small number of cells. As the tumor grows, the cancer may overpower the immune system in some individuals. This explains why some cancer patients survive, even though cancer cells have been present in their lymphatic and blood systems (their immune systems kill stray cancer cells), while others do not (their immune systems become overpowered by a virulent, aggressive cancer cell growth). (U.S. Dept. of H.H.S., 1984.)

Some researchers have emphasized that cancer seems to be a series of highly coordinated steps in which certain cells acquire unique abilities. Some tumor cells reproduce in great numbers by using a process that is used by the body to repair wounds. Cancer, in this instance, subverts a benign, healing process into a harmful one. Genes that were supposed to shut down permanently following embryonic development apparently become reactivated.

Before a cancer can begin, a complex series of unusual events must occur. The process is clearly explained for the layman in an article called *The Making of a Cancer Cell,* by Boyce Rensberger. Certain types of cancer require that **oncogenes** (or cancer cells) develop over many years from exposure to chemicals. For many persons, the disease begins with prolonged contact with **carcinogens,** such as the chemicals contained in cigarette smoke. Carcinogens undergo a molecular modification before becoming cancer-causing. Researchers at the National Cancer Institute have demonstrated that although detoxifying enzymes are expected to detoxify alien substances, in some people they inexplicably activate a harmful cancer-causing mechanism. Apparently, enzymes alter the carcinogens and this permits them to enter a cell's nucleus and bind to the

DNA. The modification just described is step 1 in a cancer-causing mutation.

Dr. Harry Gelborn of the NCI explains that clearly people differ in their susceptibility to cancer. He feels it is possible that the differences relate to the relative amounts of certain enzymes individuals have. Carcinogenic substances in certain quantities and in particular combinations, may be much more dangerous than if certain activating substances are absent (Rensberger, 1984).

Although activated carcinogens may bind to DNA, in many cases they do not. Sometimes the cell's protective mechanism prevents this from occurring. For example, scavenger molecules may easily bind to alien molecules, making them harmless. Those that elude the scavengers may harmlessly bind to proteins or other cell constituents, rather than to DNA, and even then a DNA repair mechanism may serve as a saving line of defense. The cell nucleus has special molecules that can detect abnormalities, such as alien molecules attached to genetic material. When a damaged part is cut out a new section is built from fresh DNA subunits (nucleotides). If the repair is completed before the cell divides, the cancer process is stopped. If the cell divides before the repair is completed, or if the repair procedure is faulty in some way, part of the gene affected by the bound carcinogen may be abnormally duplicated. The new cell would then inherit a mutated gene, and further cell divisions would continue to be abnormal. Even in this situation, however, cancer need not necessarily result. The carcinogen may bind to any of 50,000 genes, and most of these have no relationship to cancer. Only if the mutation occurs in certain genes is the first step toward malignancy taken (Rensberger, 1984).

Dr. Rufus Day of the NCI has said that instances of faulty DNA repair may account for up to 20 percent of human cancer cases. A single mutation, however, is probably not enough to cause cancer. When scientists have tried to induce cancer in laboratory animals, they have found that many mutations generally need to occur in the same cell that harbored the original mutation. Since there are perhaps a billion lung cells, the chances of the steps described being repeated in exactly the same sequence in the exact same cell are very small indeed. The odds increase by other processes which are still being studied. Certain chemicals, called **promoters,** increase the chances of an initiated cell's descendants (each of which carries a mutant gene) being attacked by a carcinogen, which causes a second mutation. Only after the process of mutation and promotion have gone through many cycles to accumulate just the right combinations of altered genes do the affected cells develop into a tumor.

Looking at the statistical probability of all of this, one can see why tumors take so many years to begin to develop. In studying the process we can also see why tumors are most common in body sites where cells proliferate freely, such as the skin, the uterus, and the gastrointestinal lining, but uncommon in places where tissue proliferation is rare, such as in nerve cells (Rensberger, 1984).

SPECIFIC CAUSAL FACTORS

We mentioned earlier the causes and suspected causes of cancer. A more comprehensive and specific discussion here focuses separately on the single issue of etiology.

Having explained the process and the role of promoters, it is easy to name several commonly known promoters of cancer. Cigarette tars contain both carcinogens, which initiate cells, and promoters which act on lung tissue. Saccharine and cyclamate are known to be weak carcinogens but strong promoters. Dietary fats may be promoters in the development of cancer of the breast and colon. Phenobarbitol is known to be a strong promoter of liver cells, as is estrogen of breast and uterine cells. A mechanical process, such as a knife cut, can be a promoter. When tissue is injured, cells at the site release substances that stimulate cells to proliferate more quickly to heal the wound. Although normal cells stop proliferating when the wound is closed, some initiated cells keep growing (Rensberger, 1984).

Some chemicals found in a normal diet may be able to block the cancer process in the case of chemical promoters. **Retinoids** (found in dark green and yellow vegetables) are an example of a chemical family that appears to protect against cancer.

In addition to chemical carcinogens, some cancer-producing mutations are caused by radiation damaging a DNA strand. Broken chromosomes, with pieces reattached incorrectly, may produce mutations leading to some types of cancer. The phenomenon is called **chromosome translocation** (Rensberger, 1984).

The causes of most cancers are unknown. We do know, however, that cancer is not contagious. We can also say that a bruise or an injury is not known to lead to cancer. No one food or combination of foods causes cancer, although the role of diet continues to be investigated. Known causes may be divided into four major categories: viruses, radiation, nutrition, and environmental causes. In an excellent self-education text, *Understanding Cancer,* a medical student, Mark Renneker, and a physician Steven Leib, M.D., use the research and writings of several workers to explain the primary known causes of cancer.

Viruses

A virus can be technically described as a small piece of coated nucleic acid. The nucleic acid is sometimes referred to as DNA or RNA. Throughout history viruses have been known to be quite harmful, and responsible for the start of many serious diseases, such as yellow fever, poliomyelitis, smallpox, and probably some forms of cancer. How a virus gains entry into a living cell is unknown, although several theories exist. When a cell has been invaded the virus uses the cell to produce virus proteins and virus chromosomes. It can therefore be thought of as a cell parasite. Cell transformation may occur so that the chemical, metabolic and physical changes in the cell can be observed. The new genetic materials which the virus brings to cells may then convert them into cancer cells. Cancer-causing DNA and RNA viruses are known as **oncogenic viruses.** Certain conditions must be met before scientists can, with certainty, state that a disease is definitely caused by a given infectious agent. For more than a hundred years, a series of conditions known as Koch's postulates have been used as criteria. One of Koch's criteria states that the culture must result in the same disease when it is inoculated into an animal. Since researchers cannot ethically inject potentially harmful viruses into human subjects, it is difficult to absolutely prove that a given virus causes cancer in man. Indirect proof exists, however, that suggests viral causation of some tumors. This proof is derived from experimental transmission, tissue culture, electron microscopy, and epidemiology. An example of epidemiologic proof is familial development of cancers, caused presumably by the passing from parent to child of a viral infection through germ cells (McKay, 1979).

Radiation

Although radiation is an accepted method of assessment and treatment for cancer, it is also a known cause. In its most general form, radiation may be defined as energy transmitted through space. Radiant energy takes several forms, including (1) various types of waves, such as ultra-violet light, x-rays, radiowaves, and microwaves, and (2) less well-known forms, such as atomic particles; for example, neutrons and quarks. They are all essentially tiny bits moving very rapidly through space. When persons (made up of cells) get in the way of radiation particles, there may be a collision and that individual's body could be biochemically altered. The DNA component of a cell is likely to be the most vulnerable to radiation. A change in the DNA changes the chromosomes, which could lead to a mutation resulting in cancer (Renneker and Leib, 1979).

An early example of cancer causing radiation was the tumors on the hands of people who worked with x-rays. Many animal studies have since demonstrated that radiation leads to an increase in the cancer rate. In humans radiation-induced tumors may take as long as 30 to 40 years to develop. Unlike most viral and chemical agents that cause tumors, radiation is capable of causing tumors in nearly all tissues of the body.

Leukemia is a type of cancer particularly associated with radiation. Persons exposed to the 1945 atomic explosions in Hiroshima and Nagasaki, Japan, have been extensively studied. These survivors show an increased incidence of leukemia. In the United States children whose mothers were exposed to x-rays while they were pregnant had a 40 percent higher leukemia incidence in a study done of 750,000 such cases.

Many examples of radiation leading to cancer have been cited among workers. These range from radiologists who work daily with radiation, to uranium miners in Czechoslovakia and the U.S. who were exposed to radioactive dust. A few decades ago when women were employed to paint luminous dials on watches it was observed that they developed bone tumors in large numbers. Many apparently developed a habit of licking their paint brushes, ingesting radium and other radioactive substances, which then settled in their bones (Coggle, 1971).

Nutrition

Although clues in epidemiological studies suggest that diet may be related to the formation of cancers, no absolute proof has been established. The diet-cancer interactions have not been studied carefully enough and long enough to verify relationships; consequently, the evidence must still be regarded as weak.

The average American diet consists of many foods with low levels of compounds (chemical carcinogens) which when fed to animals, cause cancer. Polycyclic aromatic hydrocarbons are chemical compounds that are strong cancer-causing substances in animals. Benzoapyrene and dibenzanthracene are the most common food contaminants. Tobacco, air pollution, and industrial exposures are more important sources of poly-cyclics than are foods. Foods containing polycyclics are smoked fish, hams, barbecued beef, cooking oils, and coffee. The strongest association has been demonstrated between smoked fish and stomach cancer. Although charring or grilling beef (thereby causing polycyclic hydrocarbons) has been linked with cancer of the bowel, there does not seem to be a clear or simple correlation. Other cofactors may be involved.

Nitrosamines are another carcinogenic found in several medicines; in addition, they are used as food preservatives. They could be associated with any type of cancer from the liver to the central nervous system. Again, there are no simple correlations. As an example, ascorbic acid is known to block nitrosamine formation. Therefore, if a person drinks a glass of orange juice before consuming bacon, perhaps he is protecting himself from the potentially harmful effects of the smoked meat. Among the Japanese, fish is a clear risk factor for stomach cancer. Salted fish contains a high level of nitrosamines. But perhaps those who consume salted fish are also eating a lot of smoked fish, and the polycyclic hydrocarbons in the latter are the real culprit.

Aflatoxins, Pesticides, Asbestos, and DES

The American food most commonly associated with aflatoxins is peanuts, and the suspected association is with liver cancer although no definitive risk has been shown. Pesticides, such as DDT, have been banned because they can produce tumors in animals, but it is not known whether pesticides are human carcinogens. Asbestos is known to be a powerful carcinogen for humans. The presence of asbestos fibers in drinking water is a major concern, and since asbestos has been used for piping, the filtration of beer, wine and soft drinks also bears watching. DES has been used to fatten cattle and chickens, and although it is not thought to be a major threat, it is a proven carcinogenic under certain conditions.

Other Suspected Dietary Risks

Carcinogens have been added to foods as a result of processing, but many potentially harmful substances are added also to foods to enhance their appearance and flavor. Dyes and artificial sweeteners are among those food additives that are highly suspect. Although animal studies have been done, with some positive results, many substances, such as cyclamates, have been in use a very short period of time; consequently, it may be too soon to determine any epidemiologic patterns of human cancer. Heavy metal—such as lead, nickel, and arsenic—are found in both food and water. They are potential carcinogens, and even though their effects may be small when compared to other risk factors, one must ask what their long-range affects may be.

No major type of cancer is common everywhere in the world. As people leave one country to settle in a second country, their cancer risks shift to that of their new country. After subtracting known cancer risk factors—for example, cigarette smoking, exposure to sunlight, sexual behaviors and working habits, a large residual of cancers are still not associated with environmental exposure or inhaled carcinogens. Therefore, these cancers are very likely attributable to diet.

People who move to the U.S. from a less affluent country increase their risk of developing bowel cancer, as well as breast, endometrial, ovarian, and prostate cancer. Persons who consume large amounts of alcohol, and who are also tobacco smokers, are at high risk for cancer of the mouth, pharynx, and esophagus (Berg, 1979).

The nutritional issue is the most controversial and publicized one today. The NCI has stated "about one-third of all cancer deaths may be related to what we eat . . . " (*Newsday*, 17 June 1987, p. 1). To inform the public about suggested dietary considerations, the NCI has published a brochure entitled *Diet, Nutrition and Cancer Prevention: The Good News.* The brochure, which was distributed free in many large supermarket chains in the latter half of 1987, advises eating certain foods more frequently and other foods less often. For example, fruits and vegetables should be added gradually to one's diet, and consumers should select low fat rather than whole milk (*Newsday*, 17 June 1987).

Environmental Causes

Dr. Irving Selikoff and Dr. E. Cuyler Hammond have studied environmental and occupational causes of cancer for more than two decades. Their work is the bedrock in this area, constituting much of what is known today about environmental causes of cancer. They presented their results at the Seventh National Cancer Conference.

According to Selikoff and Hammond, the main finding of a research study done at the Mount Sinai School of Medicine at the City University of New York in the 1970s was that 75–85 percent of cancers can be traced to environmental sources. Although it is not really known what percentage of cancer is actually attributable to environmental factors, the fact that such findings are even reported indicates a growing awareness of the environment as a major factor.

There is a long clinical latency period with most environmental causes. With few exceptions, tumors do not develop until 20 to 40 years after initial exposure to a carcinogenic agent.

Several environmental causes of cancer have been raised in earlier sections of this book. Multiple factors and cofactors need to be considered with occupational and other environmental exposures, as is the case with other etiology research. Although researchers have known for some time that occupational exposure to asbestos increases the risk of lung cancer, they subsequently learned that the risk was much greater for those asbestos workers who regularly smoked cigarettes.

Many environmental carcinogens require repeated and prolonged exposure to be dangerous. Some of the suspect environmental agents under study are talc (as found in foods and cosmetics), trace metals (foods and polluted air), benzpyrene (polluted air), carbon black (rubber tire dust), benzene (paint), PCB's (paper), DES (meats), and titanium (paints) (Selikoff and Hammond, 1979).

TREATMENTS

In general, treatments have a much better chance of success if the tumor is localized. Early diagnosis is of paramount importance. Once a tumor has metastasized, successful treatment is very difficult.

In 1900 there was essentially no cancer treatment. Forty years later, only 20 percent of patients suffering from cancer were cured. The cure rate improved to about 33 percent in the 1950s primarily due to improved surgery and radiotherapy. Today more than 40 percent of patients in this country can be cured.

Surgery

The most successful form of treatment for cancer is surgical removal of localized malignant tumors at an early stage. In later stages, surgery may be attempted in conjunction with other techniques.

The radical mastectomy is a good example of an operation, developed around the turn of the century, which greatly increases survival rates. By the end of World War I, 45 percent of women with breast cancer were declared cured. Unfortunately, the cure rate has not improved much since then. However, we now have a more sophisticated understanding of certain aspects of these operations and can predict cures more accurately. For example, if there is only a small lump in the breast and the lymph glands under the arm are not involved, the cure rate may be as high as 80 percent since it is not likely the cancer cell will shed. A lively debate continues today as to whether less-radical surgeries, such as the simple mastectomy or lumpectomy, will cure patients without psychologically or cosmetically disfiguring them and without physically disabling them, as is the case in a radical mastectomy.

In bowel cancer, surgery is still the treatment of choice. Large bowel cancer, for instance, consists of four different stages. The earliest stage— stage A—involves a very small lesion which does not invade the wall of the intestine. Shedding of cells is minimal at this stage. More than 80 percent of stage A tumors can be cured by surgery. In stage B the tumor has grown through the wall of the intestine. Surgery may still be done, but survival rate after 5 years drops to 40 to 50 percent. A stage C tumor has broken through the bowel wall and spread to the surrounding lymph glands. Surgery may still be attempted, although the outlook is not as hopeful. A stage D tumor has already metastasized.

Radiation

This common cancer treatment, sometimes referred to as radiotherapy, kills cancer cells by focusing a beam of radiation on the cancerous tissue. Cancer cells are destroyed more easily than normal cells. Radiation is usually used only when the tumor is still localized, and only if it can be used without serious radiation damage to other parts of the body. The rays may be x-rays or they may be cobalt, radium, or cesium.

The x-ray machine was developed early in the century but those in use today are greatly improved. New instruments, such as the linear accelerator, can produce megavoltage energy which provides large doses of radiation therapy to tumors with minimal damage to superficial tissues. Although radiation does kill normal cells, because of modern equipment the damage is much less permanent than in the past. Radiation, like surgery, does not attack the shed cells that are circulating in the blood; consequently, it is not effective if metastasis has occurred.

Radiation therapy alone does cure certain kinds of cancer and has contributed to an improved cancer survival rate. An example is localized cancer of the cervix which can be cured in 100 percent of the cases through radiotherapy, since the entire tumor can be encompassed.

Radiation treatment is also very valuable in the head and neck areas where surgery can be difficult as well as disfiguring. Radiation can focus on the tumor, leaving surrounding vital structures in tact.

Chemotherapy

Chemotherapy is essentially treatment by administering chemicals. The types of chemicals used are those that interfere with the reproductive processes of the cancer cells, those that interfere with the metabolic processes of the cancer cells, and those that increase the body's natural resistance to the cancer cells. Chemicals used in this way can affect the entire body, a certain region, or just the tumor. The problem with chemotherapy, however, is finding drugs that will destroy cancer cells without harming normal cells. More than 40 drugs have been developed that are useful in the treatment of certain types of cancer. In a relatively modest percentage of cases, the chemotherapy alone produces a cure; in a larger percentage of cases the chemotherapy temporarily inhibits the cancerous growth and relieves pain.

Sometimes the cancer cells multiply more rapidly than the drugs can kill them. The chemicals used are highly toxic and are not without side effects, such as reduced production of blood cells, hair loss, vomiting, diarrhea, and nausea.

One group of chemical agents, called alkylating agents, have been used with certain cancers of the lymphatic and blood forming tissues such as Hodgkin's disease, lymphosarcoma, and chronic leukemia. Another group of chemotherapeutic agents, called metabolic antagonists, are designed to starve cancer cells by interfering with their vital life processes. They are "counterfeit" materials that closely resemble those needed by cancer cells for development. They "fool" the cell into using them, resulting in a faulty cell process and a blocked activity. Methotrexate is a metabolic antagonist that has been widely used in treating acute leukemia in children.

Hormone therapy is used mainly for tumors of the endocrine glands and related organs. Hormones can be useful in treating some cancers of the breast, prostate, and uterus by changing the hormonal environment. For example, male hormones (androgens) are sometimes effective in treating young women with advanced cancer of the breast. An older woman, one past menopause, who has a breast cancer not amenable to surgery, may temporarily respond to treatment with female hormones (estrogens). Prednisone, a derivative of cortisone, is sometimes helpful with lymphoma or acute leukemia. Progesterone is used to treat endometrial cancer.

Much effort is being devoted to the search for more effective drugs to treat cancer. The National Cancer Institute has been in the forefront of this activity for decades. Each year 15,000 materials (such as chemicals, plant extracts, antibiotics, and newly synthesized compounds) are tested in rodents for anticancer activity. Those that appear promising are tested in larger animals. Some of these materials, perhaps one of every 1,000, are ultimately regarded as safe enough, and hopeful enough to be tried in humans.

Chemotherapeutic agents used in patients suffering from Hodgkins' and other lymphomas in combination are far more effective than when they are used alone. The use of effective combinations of drugs has led to very long survivals, even when the diseases are in advanced stages (Heidenstam, 1976; U.S. Dept. of H.E.W., 1978; U.S. Dept. of H.H.S., 1984).

UNPROVEN TREATMENT METHODS

In addition to the accepted treatment methods of surgery, radiation, and chemotherapy, many other approaches have been used, and are continuing to be used, to fight cancer. Some of these approaches have gained considerable acceptance and support, even among scientists. Others, however, are regarded as out-and-out fraudulent schemes to bilk desperate people. Some of the most common experimental and/or unproven treatment methods will be briefly discussed in this section.

Immunotherapy

Researchers are studying the body's natural defense system in the hopes that our own immunological system can help arrest the development of cancer. The immunological system consists of groups of cells that recognize and reject foreign substances (**antigens**). These cells produce counter substances (**antibodies**) that react with and inactivate the antigens.

Apparently some cancer tissue is antigenically different from normal tissue. Researchers hope it may be possible to mobilize body defenses against cancerous tissue. Theoretically scientists may be able to develop a vaccine made of cancer cells and use it to stimulate the production of antibodies against future cancer cells. Unfortunately, such a treatment method is not a present option.

Genetically engineered agents, called **monoclonal antibodies,** are showing promise in treating patients with stomach and colon tumors. Scientists believe monoclonal antibodies mobilize the body's immune system. Dr. Hilary Koprowski has been quoted in *U.S. News and World Report* as saying that she believes the future for immunotherapy is very bright. In Dr. Koprowski's opinion, this approach, in combination with other therapies, may make it possible to control cancer.

Innoculating patients with their own living tissue, which is prepared immediately after surgery, appears to invigorate the immune system to seek and destroy parts of the tumor that may have spread. This approach, which has been tried at the Litton Institute of Applied Biotechnology in Rockville, Maryland, has been found to slow down, and perhaps even prevent, the spread of colon cancer to other parts of the body. In a sense, this technique is **a colon cancer vaccine.** In a 1985 issue of the journal *Cancer,* physicians reported good success in a large-scale, national trial of this approach. Because so few new methods of treating cancer of the large bowel have been developed in recent years, surgical oncologists are excited with this technique (*Newsday,* 30 March 1985).

Hyperthermia

Tumor cells are heat sensitive. However, many physicians eschew heat treatment because they cannot always predict when it will work and when it will fail. When a cell is given a burst of heat exposure, it aborts all "stress proteins" that protect it from harm. This heat-shock response is regarded as an important, although still controversial, issue in cancer treatment.

About 25 years ago an Italian geneticist, Ferrucio Ritossa, discovered that specific genetic changes occurred when he inadvertently overheated a cell preparation. He published his findings, but they caused little stir at the time. Only a few years ago did Ritossa's discovery begin to generate widespread interest. The heat-shock response has been demonstrated in yeast bacteria as well as in higher animals, including humans. When a property similar to this one is shared by several species, biologists regard it as fundamental and important (*Newsday*, 8 October 1985).

David Zinman, a *Newsday* science writer, described the process. A cancer patient is placed under anesthesia. His blood is circulated from his body into a heat exchange machine and then pumped back. His temperature climbs slowly to 107 degrees and is held constant for about 4 hours. According to Dr. Nicholas Bottiglieri, Vice President for Professional Education of the American Cancer Society, at the time of the interview, hyperthermia is still in the research stage, but based on what has been seen to date, it is regarded as very promising (*Newsday*, 21 September 1981).

Varied Experimental Procedures

When facing an almost certain death sentence, many people opt to try unconventional treatments, even if the odds are long. A professor from the University of Michigan pleaded for understanding in an article first published in *The Washington Post*. He asserted that most "guinea pigs" have chosen to be subjects for experimentation, and they have been given, at the very least, a glimmer of hope. As he pointed out, "Pain and hope are better than death." The professor eloquently stated the case for experimental programs such as the large program operated by the NCI in the National Institutes of Health, located in Bethesda, Maryland (*Newsday*, 20 October 1983).

The case of a man who chose to be treated with organically grown fruits and vegetables, calf's liver, and hourly coffee enemas was the subject of a trial in the State Supreme Court of New York. A large insurance carrier refused to pay $17,000 in bills for the controversial medical treatment, which was administered in Mexico. The patient contended that he should be allowed to choose any treatment he wished, regardless of how unorthodox. The metabolic therapy he chose was first advanced in this country by the late Dr. Max Gerson in the late 1940s and has been the subject of disagreement ever since. A related question is raised by this debate: Should a health insurance company have the power of deciding the type of treatment a patient must receive in order to qualify for reimbursement?

The University of Pennsylvania's Cancer Center estimates that 10 percent of cancer patients seek unorthodox treatment. According to Dr. Sherwood Lawrence of California's Cancer Council, most medical insurers will not pay for unproven treatments; however some suits have been won by cancer patients in which reimbursement was provided for controversial treatments, including Laetrile, a drug regarded widely by U.S. physicians as ineffective (*Newsday*, 29 September 1982).

Some unusual treatments find professional supporters. A clinic operated by a doctor of zoology in the Bahamas administers a treatment which is called "immuno-augmentative therapy." Consisting of daily injections of a serum made mostly of centrifuged plasma the treatment aims to bolster the body's immunity. The Food and Drug Administration labels the clinic's director a "quack." No data has been published, so the clinic's claims can not be properly evaluated, and the Director has refused to reveal exactly what is in the serum. Some patients have praised the treatments and offer testimonials of their improvement, along with pictures of themselves looking healthy and happy. But officials who have visited the clinic feel that the serum may contain some steroids, which improve appetite and give a sense of well being as well as possibly having a temporary anti-tumor effect. The sunshine is also credited with adding to the patients' cheerfulness and their hope. The Director has stated that he has treated more than 1,700 patients, at a cost of $2,400 for the first 4 weeks of treatment and $300 a week afterward. Housing and transportation costs are additional. However, according to an FDA spokesperson, the treatment is a fraud (*Newsday*, 22 April, 1983).

Not all over-hyped, misleading, or ultimately disappointing programs or protocols are advanced by charlatans or quacks. Most failed approaches are tried by sincere, competent, and qualified medical personnel. Very often the media over-publicizes a new approach being touted as the latest "magic bullet" to kill cancer, and thousands of desperate patients who have been told they are terminal clamor to be accepted into the experimental program. A few years ago a naturally occurring substance called **interferon** was given wide publicity, and many people paid huge sums of money to be treated with it. Unfortunately, interferon proved to be a serious disappointment, and it now appears that although interferon can now be made less expensive by using genetic engineering, if it has any value for the future it will probably be in the treatment of some viral disease—but not cancer. More recently the well known Dr. Vincent

DeVita, who at the time of interview was Director of the NCI, and is currently with Memorial Sloan-Kettering, hailed **interleukin-2** as "the most promising approach to cancer at the present time." It has fallen far short of early expectations, however. Reports of a patient's death and cautionary statements by Dr. Steven Rosenberg, Director of Surgery at the NCI, followed Dr. DeVita's announcement by only one week (*Newsday,* 10 December 1985).

Gene therapy is another new approach that has caused a great stir of interest in the past few years. The experiment began by drawing bone marrow from rhesus monkeys, infecting it with a cancer virus, and re-injecting it into the monkeys' bloodstreams. With the movement to human gene therapy perhaps just around the corner, a milestone of attack on inherited disease would be reached. This approach assumes that cancer, along with many other diseases, has an inherited component. An important problem is how to get healthy genes into a patient to replace the harmful ones. The approach being tried is to use viruses as the carrying vehicle. Virologists crack open a virus, remove the harmful genes, and fill the space with the beneficial gene they want the patient to have. The virus then has the job of invading cells, carrying along its beneficial cargo. The process has been successful in mice as well as in human cells in a lab dish; however, whether or not the process will work smoothly in humans remains to be seen (*The Record,* 1 April 1986).

The NCI recently announced a new approach for screening potentially helpful anti-cancer agents. Rather than using experimental mice, substances will be screened in laboratory dishes for activity against more than 100 varieties of cancer. The new testing system, utilizing a battery of tests to screen thousands of substances with new precision, will determine more quickly and accurately which chemicals might make useful anti-cancer drugs.

Dietary Considerations in the Treatment and Prevention of Cancer

Laboratory workers have been aware for some time that tumors in animals can be affected by diet, but only recently have they explored the possibility that diet may be important in causing cancer, treating cancer, and even preventing cancer in humans. Dr. Walter Willett and Dr. Brian MacMahon did an exhaustive review of the literature on the relationship of diet and cancer, and in 1984 presented their findings in a two-part series in *The New England Journal of Medicine*. Some of their major findings follow:

> In the first major epidemiologic study relating vitamin A intake to cancer, Norwegian men whose consumption was above average had less than half the rate of lung cancer of men whose consumption was below average. Similar findings for vitamin A and lung cancer have been reported from Japan, Singapore and the U.S. and in an update of the Norwegian study. An inverse relationship has also been found between vitamin A intake and cancers of the bladder, upper gastrointestinal tract and breast.

Willett and MacMahon, 1984

Natural preformed vitamin A is found in animal source foods; beta carotene compounds are found in green and yellow vegetables. Researchers believe beta carotene compounds offer a greater protective effect than does preformed vitamin A. Not all studies support this belief, however. When an Israeli study was re-analyzed it was found that beta carotenes had no effect. Beta carotene does show a stronger protective effect when just lung cancer is considered.

Much work has been done in investigating the effects of vitamin C. The areas of England that have a low vitamin C intake have high cancer rates. Epidemiologic evidence supporting an important role for vitamin C in the prevention of cancer is minimal. Perhaps the greatest supporter of the hypothesis has been Nobel Prize winner, Linus Pauling, Ph.D. With his colleague Ewan Cameron, M.D., Dr. Pauling wrote the well-publicized book entitled *Cancer and Vitamin C,* in which some compelling evidence is presented (Cameron and Pauling, 1979). It is important to mention that Cameron and Pauling promote massive doses of vitamin C as a **treatment** for cancer (even advanced cancer)—not merely as a preventative. Willett and MacMahon admit that due to limitations of available data, one can not rule out the possibility that vitamin C is helpful.

Like vitamin C, vitamin E has received much attention as a possible effective preventative and inhibitor of cancer. Willett and MacMahon conclude, however, that relevant epidemiologic data is limited. One study showed no relation between vitamin E levels in serum samples and risk of cancer at all sites combined. Some inhibitory effect has been reported in animal studies, however. They conclude that vitamin E merits more study.

Selenium is a trace element, and it has been observed that in the

United States as well as internationally, areas with low selenium levels in the soil or in pooled blood bank serum samples have higher cancer rates than do geographic areas with higher selenium levels. The strongest data seems to be with the link between selenium and breast and colon cancer. Selenium has been shown to reduce the occurrence of some cancers in animals, and available statistics suggest some possible benefit in human beings. High levels of selenium are toxic, however.

Concerning the relationship between fiber and colon cancer, in Part 2 of Willett and MacMahon's report, they summarize international findings.

> In Norway, New York and Greece, higher ingestion of fruits and vegetables (which are major sources of fiber as well as of several vitamins) was associated with a lower risk of colon cancer. Case control studies in Israel and among American blacks have shown a protective effect of fiber. However, in a case control study among Canadians there was no such association, and Puerto Ricans with colon cancer actually reported greater fiber intake than did controls.

> Willett and MacMahon, 1984

Although the available epidemiologic data is not consistent, generally the weight of evidence supports the theory that fiber protects against colon cancer.

There is some evidence that diets high in fat increase the risk of colon cancer, and it has been suggested that high-fat, low-fiber diets act synergistically. Although national incidence rates and per capita consumptions of fats are very strongly associated, studies of individual subjects do not provide consistent data.

Although relationship between a high intake of fats and breast cancer has been hypothesized; it is far from being proven. Greater weight has also been associated with breast cancer; consequently, excessive calories are also being examined as a causative factor.

Overall, information about specific dietary factors is inconsistent and incomplete. According to Willett and MacMahon, evidence is not strong enough to make specific dietary recommendations. They do believe, however, that the recommendations made by the National Research Council—that people should eat more fruits, vegetables, and whole grains, and less fat, and that they should use alcohol and processed foods in moderation—can certainly do no harm, and that they might be even beneficial in preventing other diseases (Willett and MacMahon, 1984).

Macrobiotic Diets

Considerable recent publicity, especially in connection with the AIDS health crisis, has been given to the macrobiotic diet. But even before AIDS became prevalent, many cancer patients were trying macrobiotic diets. It was first promoted in the U.S. by George Oshawa, who lectured on Zen macrobiotic diets in the 1960s. The most restrictive macrobiotic diet consists entirely of cereals; the least restrictive one has the following distribution of foods: 10 percent cereals, 30 percent cooked vegetables, 10 percent soup, 30 percent animal meats, 15 percent fruits and salads, and 5 percent desserts. The Council of Foods and Nutrition of the American Medical Association condemns the more restrictive diets because of their nutritional inadequacies, and warns that many illnesses may result from strict adherence to them.

Michio Kushi is the founder and president of the East West Foundation, and has spoken widely on macrobiotic diets. He also founded a company that distributes macrobiotic food. Kushi states that cancer is the result of improper diet, improper thinking, and improper lifestyle. He has many recommendations on what to eat, when to eat and how to chew food, as well as recommendations on cooking methods, sleep, clothing, house-keeping, bathing, and exercise. Kushi regards conventional treatments, such as chemotherapy, radiation, and surgery, as "violent or artificial." There is no scientific evidence nor documentation to date that macrobiotic diets are effective treatments for cancer. The only evidence of cures consists of testimonials (*Ca-A Cancer Journal for Clinicians*, 1984).

Open Minded Skepticism

The American Cancer Society maintains an official list of unproven cancer treatments. This list includes laetrile (ground-up apricot pits), chaparral tea, and the "grape cure." Sometimes substances are removed from the list and move up to a position of greater respect, although this is rare. For example, hydrazine sulfate (HS), a chemical used to kill insects, clean boilers, and fuel rockets, was on the ACS list until 1979. A study at the Syracuse Cancer Research Institute suggested that HS may help some cancer patients by altering their metabolism. Although HS is not thought to cure cancer, there is some evidence that it can help patients with advanced cancer conserve energy, gain weight, and better withstand the rigors of chemotherapy or surgery (Seligmann, 1983).

As human service workers hear clients talk hopefully of new and promising treatments, they need to keep in mind that open-minded skepticism is probably the best posture when dealing with unproven treatments. Very often in medicine, when one event follows another closely in time, the first event is assumed to be responsible for the second. This fallacious reasoning can be very dangerous, very harmful, and very expensive. Many patients and many panicked families have flown to distant places to purchase expensive chemicals and other agents in the hopes of changing a terminal diagnosis. It must be remembered that, according to experienced clinicians, in about 10 percent of all cancer cases spontaneous, unexplained remissions take place but these remissions are temporary. Many unproven treatment substances (such as Krebiozen, a cancer treatment promoted about 30 years ago by a Yugoslav physician named Steven Durovic) claim an approximate 11 percent rate of temporary benefit. Thus, short-term improvement is seen in about the same number of cases as would occur with no therapy at all (Feinberg, 1985).

Discussion in this section on treatments has been limited to medical and dietary approaches. Other interventions—such an self-healing through meditation, self-hypnosis, visualization, exercise, positive thinking, and lowering stress levels—have received considerable attention in recent years. They are not, however, regarded by most objective observers as "treatment" methods. Rather, they may be viewed as a sort of self-help, or a self-counseling aid, or a form of support to be used in conjunction with other, more conventional, treatments. They will be discussed in that context more fully in a later section.

SITES OF CANCER

Cancers grow nearly everywhere in the body. Some of the most common sites are the skin, breasts, lungs, colon and rectum, prostate, uterus, stomach, esophagus, and liver. Frequency varies among countries, and between the sexes. For example, while cancer of the liver (as the primary site) is very common in Nigeria and cancer of the stomach has high prevalence in Japan, these are uncommon primary sites in the United States.

In its booklet *Cancer Facts and Figures*, the American Cancer Society discusses each of the most common forms of cancer. These are summarized below.

Lung Cancer

For decades lung cancer has been among the most common cancer sites for men but in recent years the lung cancer death rate for women has risen alarmingly, having surpassed breast cancer in prevalence. Lung cancer is a very deadly form of cancer. Only about 13 percent of diagnosed lung cancer patients survive five years. Warning signals include a persistent cough, blood in the sputum, recurrent bronchitis and pneumonia, and chest pain. The greatest risk factor is cigarette smoking. Exposure to certain industrial substances, such as asbestos, which was mentioned earlier, is also a factor, especially for smokers.

Lung cancer is difficult to diagnose early. When smokers quit, early cellular changes in a damaged bronchial lung may return to normal. If smoking continues, however, abnormal cellular growth progresses to cancer. The chest x-ray, the sputum cytology test, and the fiberoptic bronchoscope help diagnose lung cancer.

Treatment modalities include surgery, radiation treatment, and chemotherapy, but in most cases surgery is the treatment of choice. Radiation and chemotherapy are often used in addition to surgery because the tumor frequently spreads.

Breast Cancer

Breast cancer is very common in women, and may occur in men, although rarely. Warning signals are in the breast—changes such as lumps, thickening, swelling, puckering, dimpling, skin irritation, or a scaliness or distortion of the nipples. There may also be tenderness, pain in the nipples, or discharge. Risk factors include a personal or family history of breast cancer, having had a first child after 30, or never bearing children.

The American Cancer Society recommends regular self-examination of the breasts. For women at high risk, and women over 50 years of age, a mammography is recommended annually. Professional breast exams should be done periodically after the age of 20, increasing to annual exams by the age of 40.

Treatment should include surgery when a curable tumor is diagnosed. The surgery might be simple removal of the lump with some adjuvant breast tissue (**lumpectomy**), removal of the entire breast (**total mastectomy**) removal of the entire breast and auxilliary lymph nodes (**modified**

radical mastectomy) removal of the entire breast, auxilliary lymph nodes and underlying muscles (**radical mastectomy**).

Radiation and chemotherapy may also be recommended.

Colorectal Cancer

Colorectal cancer is very common in both men and women. Warning signals include frequent rectal bleeding and changes in bowel habits, such as diarrhea or constipation, or alternating diarrhea and constipation.

Risk factors are a personal or family history of polyps in the bowels or of ulcerative colitis. Some researchers believe that bowel cancer may be related to dietary factors. Diets high in beef and diets deficient in fiber or bulk are being investigated as possible causes.

A digital rectal exam should be performed by a physician each year after the age of 40, according to the American Cancer Society. A stool guaiac slide test is a way of testing feces for hidden blood. This test is recommended annually after the age of 50, or before 50 if there is a personal history of colorectal cancer.

In a **proctosigmoidoscopy** exam the physician can examine the rectum and lower colon with the use of a hollow, lighted tube. A **flexible sigmoidoscopy** allows the physician to inspect more of the bowel. With a **colonoscopy** the entire colon can be viewed; tissue may also be biopsied. A significant number of colorectal cancers can be detected with the use of these instruments. It is recommended that persons have two yearly exams with a "procto" after age 50; if the results of these exams are negative, the patient should request a re-examination every 3 to 5 years.

When a tumor in the bowel is present, surgery is the most effective treatment. Radiation and adjuvant chemotherapy may also be used. If the surgery prevents two ends of the bowel from being resected, a **stoma** (an opening in the abdominal wall) must be made so body waste can be eliminated. The procedure is called a **colostomy**; it may be either temporary or permanent.

Skin Cancer

Although skin cancer is one of the most common forms of cancer it is also the least dangerous. Most skin cancers are highly curable **basal** or **squamous** cell cancers. There is a very serious form of skin cancer, however, that must be detected and treated quickly. This skin cancer is called **malignant melanoma** and often appears as a mole or darkly pigmented growth.

Most skin cancers are known to be caused by exposure to the sun; specifically, overexposure to the sun's ultraviolet rays. Other risk factors include a fair complexion and occupational exposure to coal tar, creosote, arsenic, and radium.

Basal and squamous cell cancers often appear as pale, waxy modules or a reddish, scaly patch. Melanomas are nearly always brown or black in appearance and they may increase in size, bleed easily, and change color.

Prevention of skin cancer includes using sunscreen preparations while exposed to the sun, wearing protective clothing, and avoiding the hours when ultraviolet rays are the strongest (10 a.m. to 3 p.m.).

Treatment for skin cancer includes surgery, radiation, tissue destruction by heat or freezing, or a combination of these. About 95 percent of patients with basal cell and squamous cell cancers have a 5-year survival rate. Malignant melanoma metastasizes quickly, however, and the 5-year survival rate for white patients with this more deadly form of skin cancer is 80 percent. If the melanoma has spread by the time of treatment, the rate of survival is 46 percent.

Oral Cancer

Heavy use of tobacco and alcohol are risk factors for oral cancer. Men are afflicted with this type of cancer much more frequently than women. Any part of the oral cavity may be affected, including the mouth, tongue, throat, and lip.

Danger signals include a sore that doesn't heal; a sore that bleeds easily; a lump or thickening; a persistent reddish or whitish patch; and difficulty in chewing, swallowing, and moving the tongue or jaws.

Abnormal tissue can be identified in regular dental check-ups. Surgery and radiation are the most common forms of treatment. Survival rates vary from less than 32 percent for cancer of the pharynx to nearly 91 percent for lip cancer.

Leukemia

Many people have the perception of leukemia as a childhood disease, but actually far more adults are stricken than children.

Leukemia is a cancer of the blood forming tissues. Causes of most cases are unknown, but some heredity linkage has been established, and exposure to radiation and certain chemicals is thought to be causal in some cases. A biopsy of bone marrow and blood tests are needed to establish the diagnosis.

In children, leukemia strikes suddenly with cold-like symptoms, and progresses quickly. Lymph nodes and the liver are enlarged; the child may appear pale and complain of fatigue. Weight loss, nose bleeds, and repeated infections are other symptoms.

Chemotherapy has been the most effective treatment. Overall survival rate is not good for this disease—28 percent for black patients and 33 percent for white patients. There has been great improvement in the treatment of lymphocytic leukemia in children, however. Twenty-five years ago leukemia was nearly always fatal, but today up to 75 percent of the children stricken with leukemia are alive or past the 5-year mark (American Cancer Society, 1987).

INCIDENCE AND PROGRESS

Figures detailing incidence rates as well as treatment success rates are tricky and difficult to summarize. Much conflicting material is presented, and the conclusions drawn are not always clearly supportable. Some of the data presented in periodicals and newspapers, at conferences, and by research and service organizations does not seem to agree.

The American Cancer Society published a booklet some time ago entitled *The Hopeful Side of Cancer.* It offers hope and encouragement, and is written in an upbeat, positive tone. The booklet begins by saying: "Cancer is one of the most curable of the major diseases in this country." Survival rates quoted are 1 in 5 by the late 1930s; 1 in 4 by the 1940s; and 1 in 3 by 1975. It is further asserted that the statistics could improve to 1 in 2 if the disease were detected early and treated immediately. The importance of early detection is discussed in the context of available diagnostic procedures.

Pap Test. Deaths from uterine cancer are declining. The death rate from this form of cancer dropped 65 percent from 1935 to 1975. The pap test reveals cancers that develop in the cervix (neck of the uterus) and the endometrium (body of the uterus).

Endometrial Detection. Although the pap test is 100 percent effective in detecting cervical cancer, it reveals only about 60 percent of endometrial cancers. Newer techniques, including removing samples of tissues from the uterus, increase detection rates.

Colorectal Detection. As discussed in an earlier section, the procto-sigmoidoscope was a great aid in detecting polyps and tumors in the rectum and lower colon. Cancers of the colon and rectum were the most common form of serious cancer in this country at the time *The Hopeful Side of Cancer* was written. Lung cancer has since become more common. Skin cancer hits more Americans than either colorectal or lung cancer, but a much greater number of people are easily treated and cured of most skin cancers. The colonoscopy, which allows the entire lower bowel to be examined, and the occult blood in stool test, which uses guaiac treated paper slides, are fairly new advances credited with detecting colon and rectal cancers at earlier stages.

Breast Self-Exam. Although 80 percent of breast lumps are non-cancerous, regular breast self-examination is an effective early warning system.

Mammography. A low radiation x-ray of the breast can reveal a tumor too small to be detected by physical exam.

Thermography. Abnormalities of the breast raise the temperature of the area. This device measures the heat patterns of the skin of the breast.

Emphasis on Prevention. The American Cancer Society has, especially in the last decade, widely emphasized prevention, and publicized steps people can take to lower the risk of developing cancer. Quitting cigarette smoking and limiting exposure to the sun have been emphasized among the preventative measures that could have a profound effect on the cancer rate. The warning signs that the American Cancer Society stresses are:

- Change in bowel or bladder habits,
- A sore that does not heal,
- Unusual bleeding or discharge,
- Thickening or lump in breast or elsewhere,
- Indigestion or difficulty in swallowing,
- Obvious change in wart or mole,
- Nagging cough or hoarseness.

In its publication *Cancer Facts and Figures,* the American Cancer Society explains the difficulty getting accurate cancer data. Cancer is not a reportable disease in most states. Estimates used to be drawn from a few cancer registries, and by the late 1960s the National Cancer Institute had started a major 3-year study of incidence, utilizing nine major population centers in the U.S. NCI expanded that effort in the mid-70s. It sometimes seems that sharp changes in health data warn of an epidemic or hint of a successful treatment or cure, but it most frequently is simply a change in data base as new incidence information becomes available.

In the early part of this decade, much-improved cure rates were being reported. A cure is generally defined as survival for 5 years after treatment with no sign of the disease remaining. Advances in chemotherapy were generally credited for the improved cure rates. By late 1981 an overall 40 percent cancer cure rate was being claimed, which represented an improvement of 25 percent over 1950 survival rates. Childhood leukemia, Hodgkins disease, and testicular cancer were among the types of cancer that were more successfully treated (Clark et al., 1981). In 1982 the American Cancer Society began a major epidemiological study involving one million Americans. Thousands of volunteers were drafted to gather information about the health and life styles of their friends and acquaintances. The study, still underway, hopes to discover environmental factors and traits of life style that may give people cancer, or protect them from it. The volunteers check back on their subjects every 2 years. Researchers have examined many areas including diet; passive smoking; low-tar and low-nicotine cigarettes; certain prescription medications, such as oral contraceptives; tranquilizers; and hormones. Long-term exposure to low levels of radiation; the effects of air and water pollution; and possible racial, religious, and geographic links with cancer are additional areas that are being examined with computer assistance.

In late 1983 Dr. DeVita, then Director of the National Cancer Institute, was quoted in *The Washington Post* as reporting a 50 percent overall cancer survival rate. Dr. DeVita credited slow, steady progress for the improvements. He noted that there are now 10 times as many oncologists as there were in 1970. Dr. DeVita based his estimate on reports from leading cancer centers. Although their cure rates generally run about 15 percent higher than nationwide rates, it is thought that the rest of the country will eventually catch up to these leaders. In recent years there has been debate about using the term "cure rate" synonymously with the 5-year survival rate since some cancers—for example, breast, kidney, and prostate cancer—can recur many years later. About 85 percent of those cancer patients who survive the first 5 years will be alive in another 5 years (Cohn, 1983).

Some evidence that an adverse socioeconomic background may have a negative effect on cancer survival was suggested by a study completed at Harlem Medical Center. According to Dr. David Savage, a stressful environment, such as overcrowded living conditions, was as important in predicting survival as was clearly defined clinical factors, such as tumor size (*Newsday*, 17 April, 1986).

The poor are not the only group at special risk for developing cancer; the elderly also have increased risk. With the graying of America, there is sure to be an increased number of cancer-susceptible people during the next several decades. No one knows for sure why the elderly are particularly at risk. Some experts feel it may be due to many years of continued exposure to carcinogens, combined with a gradual weakening of the body's immune system. Government officials estimate that by the year 2030 there will be as many as 65 million people 65 years of age and older. Age is simply the greatest risk factor for all cancers (*Newsday*, 29 April 1986).

The roller coaster of cancer hopefulness took a sharp rise in November 1986 when Dr. Eric T. Fossel of Boston's Beth Israel Hospital reported on a new blood test that appears to accurately detect all forms of cancer. The test uses nuclear magnetic resonance to reveal differences in the magnetic properties of the blood plasma of cancer patients. Such a test may some day provide a simple means of routinely screening people for cancer.

Cancer patients and health professionals both agree that although the picture is not all bright, there are many reasons for hopefulness. This is a very active time. Cancer has received high media attention and, as a result, the public is interested. Years ago it was a taboo subject, but today people speak openly about cancer. We are on the doorstep of major change. There is great vitality and interest and this is good news for those who have waited as well as those who are waiting for the ultimate answer in preventing, detecting, treating, and curing this most dreaded health foe.

Chapter 5

COUNSELING PERSONS WITH CANCER

Now that the counseling process has been discussed and a primer for understanding cancer has been provided, an attempt will be made to relate these two bodies of knowledge. This section might have been better entitled "Counseling **and** Persons with Cancer" so the interactive nature of the process would be emphasized. To speak only of "counseling a person" implies that a process is being done **to** someone, that the person is receiving some knowledge or understanding. Although that is often the case, we need to allow for many of the other experiences that counseling opens up. As discussed in the earlier sections on the counseling process, expressing and acknowledging feelings should be a major part of all types of counseling. Counseling need not be done **to** a client or a patient or a counselee, and it need not be done **by** a fully trained counselor or a therapist or any other professional human services worker. Peer counseling, a totally legitimate form of assistance, even when the counselor has few formal qualifications, is becoming a prevalent form of counseling, especially among persons with disabilities. Another form of counseling is when clients advise each other informally in various types of support groups. Although not counseling **per se,** gaining understanding (and possibly acceptance of one's condition or feelings) by reading books, booklets, leaflets, and other written materials might be regarded as a pre-counseling, or counseling-related, activity. The major drawback here, of course, is the lack of interaction. Nonetheless, reading booklets that offer advice may be the only resource available to some people or the only resource they're receptive to. Booklets may encourage an individual to seek out a counselor, and prepare him for the counseling experience.

The point is that counseling comes in many forms, and the counselor could be a patient/client or he could be a trained professional. The setting might be a physician's office or donated space in a church basement. The counseling might be a single session as part of another process (for example, in conjunction with medical information supplied by a health professional) or it might be a long-term process (for example, psychoanalytic therapy).

The objective of the counseling might be to alleviate a general feeling of depression, or it might have a very specific short-term goal, such as counseling the individual on re-employment rights or vocational options in view of physical limitations. A process that begins with a limited, specific goal might be broadened as new feelings and problems come to light. The need for more extensive counseling might become apparent only after the client becomes committed to, and comfortable with, the process.

EMOTIONAL STATE OF THE PERSON WITH CANCER

It seems fairly evident that a cancer diagnosis would be a devastating blow for most people. Dr. Bernie Siegel writes of a patient who, as soon as she learned she had cancer, donated all her clothes to Goodwill Industries, a clear giving-up action. Most people who are informed they have this dreaded disease overflow with emotion. Dr. Siegel believes that denial is universally used at first, and that this allows for gradual acceptance. Depression occurs, but it may be delayed by months, because this is when the patient really hears what he has been told. Dr. Siegel has seen some people who have acted close to psychotic in an almost total denial. Withdrawal from human contact is common, and a feeling of despair may continue for months, even years.

Self-pity and "Why me?" are other common reactions cited by Dr. Siegel, and familiar to those who have worked with persons who have cancer. Anger is often felt, but not usually expressed against the cigarette industry, the pesticide industry, the food additive industry, the nuclear power industry, or any other industry that may be partially responsible. Rage is often felt toward God, toward one's self, or toward family members who are perceived as having made the patient unhappy and therefore driven to self-destructive behavior, such as smoking.

Some patients have strong guilt feelings. They blame themselves for having done something directly causitive, or, in a more general way, they condemn themselves for having been bad and feel they are being punished (Siegel, 1986).

A major study of the non-medical problems and the needs of cancer patients who survive was undertaken by the California Division of the American Cancer Society. Interviews were conducted two to three years after the initial cancer diagnosis. By that time most patients had stabilized and did not appear highly stressed. But some continued to be depressed years after their diagnosis. Intermittent attacks of deep depression occurred especially at night or when they were alone. Suicide was sometimes mentioned. Some patients reported delayed reactions of approximately six months after they were diagnosed before they experienced fits of depression, and sometimes bouts of heavy drinking. The key periods of stress were right before the diagnosis (when they were awaiting their test results), when they were actually diagnosed, and when they were hospitalized (American Cancer Society, California Division, 1979).

SOME COMMON EMOTIONS AND STAGES

The writer has counseled many persons with cancer since becoming affiliated in 1981 with a New York program serving the needs of cancer patients. It should be mentioned, perhaps, that he is himself a cancer survivor. Although he has been a trained counselor for many years, his cancer experience was the primary motivator for embarking on this new specialty area.

The counseling has ranged from a limited number of meetings about specific issues and defined in advance by the client, to long-term counseling relationships lasting years and covering virtually all aspects of personal adjustment and vocational issues. In addition to this core group of counselees, many family members and friends have become "adjunct counselees." Scores of phone contacts and brief in-person interactions, such as those that occur at group meetings, have added to the writer's fabric of understanding and experience. Since his own diagnosis and recovery from cancer, the writer has encountered, observed, listened to, and interacted with several hundred persons with cancer at meetings, rap groups, and training conferences. Several areas of common experience have emerged. Some persons seem to go through stages; others report only one or two conscious emotions connected with the experience. Not all persons experience all stages, nor are the stages necessarily in the order they are presented here. But when all the stages are present, they usually occur in the order described below.

Fear. Hearing the words, "You have cancer" nearly always provokes a fear reaction. It is natural and normal that it should. Cancer has been feared for centuries, and many people still think of it as an absolute death sentence.

Shock. Many persons report a classic shock reaction. Not understanding or being able to process information, especially medical information, is a frequently reported early stage. "I just walked around in a daze for weeks" is a typical statement by a person looking back to when he was diagnosed.

Disbelief. Persons with cancer often describe the doubt they experienced upon learning of their diagnosis. Checking and double checking with physicians is common. Because the information seems so unreal and so unbelievable, the defense of denial is commonly employed. I called the radiology clinic a few days after receiving my cancer diagnosis "just to be sure." I recalled hearing a technician mention that another man with the same surname had been in for x-rays that morning. "Of course, it must be a mistake; that other man has the cancer—not me" was my reaction. The secretary calmly and convincingly explained that the other gentleman had had a completely different series of x-rays and that a mixup was impossible. Boing! Back to reality. For some patients, the process of disbelief never occurs; for others it lasts much longer.

Confusion and Distractibility. Often accompanying fear, shock, and disbelief, patients are unable to concentrate, to remember, to do things that require judgment. Making decisions seems to require the use of too much energy for people who feel energy-depleted. Doing things by rote, or "going through the motions" in household chores or work-related routines, is the way many recently diagnosed cancer patients describe their activities. Nearly everyone with cancer reports being distracted at least some of the time, even if it's as mild as occasional "daydreaming." Patients who are hard-hit by the cancer diagnosis are often unable to function at work, especially when their job is complex, at least until a recovery stage has been reached.

Depression. The most widespread and universal emotion for persons dealing with cancer is depression. The depression is not feeling "just a little blue"; rather it ranges from moderate to severe. It typically perseveres for months, and very often requires professional intervention. Some patients do not recognize they are depressed. Even families and friends may fail to recognize the symptoms. The person may simply appear to have become thoughtful, pensive, or quiet.

Altruism. A surprising number of persons move out of their depression (or out of their initial depression) into an upbeat, hopeful, altruistic phase that can be described as a "help the world syndrome." Many patients, as they are mending medically, plan to begin some human service activities when they recover. In a way it appears to be a thankful gesture for having made it through the early stages of the illness and the treatment process. In a different view, however, it appears to be a bargaining with God, an offer to do some good for humanity with a life that has taken on new meaning and preciousness.

Falling Apart. Too often the hopeful, altruistic, frenzied-planning stage is quickly followed by a feeling of helplessness and panic. A new surge of fear may occur. This new fear often centers on the cancer recurring. Previously the fear may have been focused on surviving a surgery, or perhaps on a generalized fear of the whole situation. This new stage is a fertile one for therapeutic intervention. Persons experience extreme emotions at this time, often complicated by phobias and other pre-morbid dysfunctions which have re-emerged or which, in some cases, have been allowed to surface for the first time. The helplessness and vulnerability often lead persons to seek professional counseling. Physically stronger, with the cancer under control, the person wants to increase his chances of staying well by understanding the whole cancer experience.

Acceptance. In this stage many persons accept the fact that the unthinkable can, and did, happen to them. Their thoughts waiver: I got cancer-...but I'm still alive...many things in life are the same...but some things look and feel different...why me?...why not me?...what can I do now about keeping cancer away from my door?...maybe not much... perhaps there are a few things worth trying. Persons who are terminal or who are uncertain about their prognosis may also experience the acceptance phase. In some cases, acceptance means not only accepting the cancer, but accepting impending death. Peacefulness and calmness characterize the acceptance stage, although the peace and calm are not always permanent. Patients who become cancer survivors of long-standing sometimes report that returning to the hustle-bustle of daily cares, work, and worries gradually erodes the peacefulness and the calmness they felt for months or years.

Normalcy. Newly diagnosed patients find it hard to believe that they will not be obsessed forever with the fact that cancer has invaded their body. Slowly, gradually, with time and with physical and psychic healing, normalcy returns. Perhaps some of the peacefulness is gone, but so is the intense fear. Some of the altruism has been forgotten, but the period of time between thoughts about cancer gradually increases from hours to days to weeks. The victim or martyr or saint recedes, and the person reemerges, often with a new and healthy dimension.

Some patients do not survive long enough to go through all of these stages. With certain clients, several of these phases are not seen. A few of the phases, such as the altruism stage, are limited to a rather small percentage of people.

It is hoped that counselors will have their awareness heightened by this discussion so they will be able to recognize some of these stages and know that they are common, natural, and transient. Persons with cancer may also find some solace in seeing themselves, to one degree or other, in the descriptions of these stages, knowing that with time, motivation, a little luck and perhaps some professional intervention the disturbing cluster of feelings need not cling on forever.

FAMILY REACTIONS

In a California study, carried out by Greenleigh Associates and published by the California Division of the American Cancer Society, considerable data was gathered about family reactions and feelings. Family members, like patients, blamed physicians and other medical personnel for the high stress they were experiencing. They felt they were entitled to more information. As might be expected, the most stressful period for families of terminal patients was when they learned of the impending death of their relative.

When family members were asked if patients fully understood their health condition, nearly 90 percent said they did. This is a major change that has gradually occurred over the past several decades. Family members have told researchers that other relatives and friends had generally been a very positive factor during the patient's illness. Most patients and their families also said no social services were made available to them. Both groups expressed a need for the services and more information about cancer. The service made most available was visits from clergy. Both patients and their families felt that more support was needed from medical personnel in times of crises, and that attention should be directed to the special needs of children. The family members of deceased patients expressed a need for support and service (American Cancer Society, California Division, 1979).

None of the findings of the Greenleigh Associates study regarding family members' reactions was particularly surprising to the writer.

These are reports and complaints commonly heard by workers in the field. One finding, however, does merit attention: a high percentage of relatives reported that their loved one was highly aware of his/her health condition. This is an encouraging, positive sign, but it might be somewhat exaggerated. A probing interviewer might have elicited this statement from a spouse: "Well I know he knew. We never mentioned the word 'cancer,' but I'm sure he must have discussed those things with his doctor." In other words, the family may have assumed that the patient was fully aware of the severity of his condition, but no attempt was made by the researchers to verify this.

Family members appear, in some cases, to be as stressed as the patients themselves; in other cases, even more so. The patient is dealing with, and is forced to cope with, his situation. The caring relative must often stand by helplessly, feeling impotent and frustrated.

The California study stresses spouses as "family," but the importance of childrens' reactions should not be overlooked. A number of concerned adult children also seek support and counseling. And, in several cases, children have been the referral source for counseling, seeking information and help when the patient's spouse is unable to do so for him/herself. While the spouse may act devastated and withdrawn and feel inadequate in dealing with medical and social services personnel, an energized child will often fill in the gap, making arrangements for the ill parent, dealing with professionals, and seeking personal advice and comfort. This occurs when marriages are intact as well as when there has been divorce. It might be a mature single young adult, or a married older child who is juggling the responsibilities and worries of two families. A spouse, a parent or an adult child will, in some cases, seek to protect a loved one by withholding information and asking others to do likewise. Professionals have often acceeded to such requests, feeling perhaps that it was a spouse's "right" or a parent's "duty" to spare pain and suffering. Many professionals have not faced their own fears about cancer, or about death, and these fears tend to cloud their thinking and distort their judgment. Often it is simply the path of least resistance. It is much easier for a physician to agree to withhold medical information from a patient than to take the time to attempt changing the family's attitude. A common theme among self-help books is that a positive attitude is essential in having the strength and energy necessary to fight life's adversities. Therefore, family members often withhold or distort information because they feel that giving discouraging news to a patient will somehow cause him "to lose hope." There is much food for thought in these assertions, and some compelling data has been presented to back up this claim. It has never been proven, however, that mental attitude is in any way related to developing or recovering from cancer. Much of the advice offered in such books is fine and it may be useful for some people, but we must also think of the negative consequences that can result when the patient is under the impression that he caused his cancer, or that he nurtures it. The guilt and discouragement may be far more psychically dangerous and energy-depleting than if his medical situation had been explained to him sensitively and truthfully.

TYPES OF COUNSELING NEEDS

Medical information

After recovering from the initial shock of hearing he has cancer, the person requires medical information and advice. Cancer patients report that they fail to "hear" much of what is said to them in early meetings with their physicians. Medical personnel need to be aware of this fact. It may be necessary to repeat and clarify the same information many times over. The shock of what is happening to him and the anxiety he is experiencing may be interfering with the patient's ability to process and analyze the material he's receiving. Clients report that when they take someone with them to conferences with doctors and compare notes afterward they find that the calmer friend or relative often hears and remembers information that they have missed.

A person may learn that he has cancer as a result of routine screening examinations at work or at a community health project. Wide-scale and routine screening is a good thing, and more of it needs to be done. A major disadvantage, however, is that the medical personnel performing the examinations are usually strangers to the patient. Such emotionally charged material is better shared by a person who has a relationship with the patient.

A general screening program may just point to a potential problem, without confirming a diagnosis. In such cases, a patient may be referred to his own doctor for further testing. Some people do not have a "family doctor," however. In such cases it is imperative for the health screening team to provide a specific referral to a qualified physician or laboratory, and then to follow-through to be certain the patient made an appointment and kept it. A follow-up phone call is advisable in all cases where cancer (or other serious illness) is suspected, even when the patient seems reliable and says he will make an appointment with his own physician. The writer counseled a bright, professional man who had become immobilized with fear upon learning from a large and reputable screening clinic in New York City that he might have a serious health problem. He delayed following through with further examinations for several months, seriously jeopardizing his health. Fortunately, the tumor was still operable and the client recovered, but that was a bit of luck that should not be relied on. The screening clinic was impersonal and not the least bit apologetic when told that their negligence in following up could have cost the patient his life. The clinic maintained that follow-through is the patient's responsibility, and that they see too many patients to check to see whether each does, in fact, seek further examination.

Suspected cancer must be handled with the utmost care and sensitivity. The seriousness of the situation must be conveyed to the patient without alarming him to such a degree that he is shocked into inaction or total denial. A family doctor might refer the patient to a specialist, such as an oncologist or a surgeon, who must take the time to talk to the patient. This is often the first type of advice, guidance, or support—the first counseling—that a patient receives. The specialist might find it convenient to assume that the referring health care worker had already discussed the matter with his patient, and this could be the case. But the patient needs to receive information, support, and reassurance at every turn. He has a tremendous need to hear what can be done for him, and to have the positives clearly spelled out. If a patient is not told that treatments have a good chance of arresting the cancer, he will assume there is no hope. Without providing an overly optimistic picture, the patient needs to be assured that everything possible will be done for him medically. His options must be clearly spelled out.

Sometimes there are specialty hospitals, cancer centers, or experimental programs that might provide a greater hope for successful treatment. If so, this information needs to be provided. The patient probably has neither the clarity of mind nor the energy to search out these options or to consider their pros and cons. Patients sometimes select a hospital simply because it is close to home and easy for relatives to visit. Although patients should see caring people during serious illness, this is not the only, and certainly not the most important, consideration. That point of view may need to be expressed to the patient for his consideration. When the medical prognosis is bleak, physicians and nurses become even "busier," and the likelihood increases that the patient will not receive much information. All people experiencing health problems have a right to know the nature of their problem and what the future may hold for them. Even patients who are terminally ill can derive comfort from talking frankly with sensitive medical personnel. For example, patients are often tremendously relieved to hear that pain control medication is available and that it will be freely administered. Many persons do not know this and spend many worried hours in fear of their last days when they imagine they will be in unbearable pain.

Cancer patients, and their advocates, should assure that the level of pain control medication is appropriate. In this country there is some hesitancy about use of some pain control substances, such as heroin. In nearly 50 other countries—including England, Spain, Australia, and Belgium—heroin is often used in combination with other drugs to relieve the pain of terminal cancer. There is a natural hesitation to legitimize a substance that has a vast illegal market, but nonetheless a movement is underway to legalize heroin for control of intractable pain; several bills toward that end have been introduced in the U.S. Congress. Needless to say, strict safeguards would clearly need to be put in place to prevent heroin from being diverted into illegal channels.

Although not as effective as heroin, there are many other strong pain-reducing medications which U.S. physicians can, and do, legally prescribe. Patients need to be forthright in dealing with medical personnel to assure that they die with dignity. No one needs to die in agony. A patient can spell out his wishes in a "living will," or in a frank discussion with his physicians while he is still feeling well. The patient, for whatever reason, may have failed to make his wishes known to his doctor when lucid, and then becomes too ill to communicate. It may then be up to his relatives to provide comfort.

Although medical personnel probably regard their health care skills as their sole qualification, they may, with practice, develop formidable counseling skills. Even without formal training, bright and sensitive people who are repeatedly thrown into situations where communication, understanding, and relating are critical may, through trial and error, learn the rudiments of good counseling. Feeling inadequate in these circumstances, some nurses, but few physicians, study counseling formally. Because nurses in strictly medical settings have limited power to assist patients, they sometimes "burn out." They find they prefer the interactive part of their work with patients over the more technical health care aspects.

In recent years many nurses have become nurse-therapists, with formal training in psychotherapeutic techniques. Some counsel in hospital settings, but an increasing number have been establishing private practices in psychotherapy. They bring with them, of course, great knowledge and experience which can be combined with their newly developed skills and talents. Consequently, nurse-therapists are often found specializing in the therapeutic touch, a sort of specialized massage and bio-feedback technique whereby the patient is taught to control certain bodily functions—such as skin temperature, breathing rate, and blood pressure—by seeing the indices of these on machines, as he practices behavioral relaxation exercises.

Reflexology—a belief that massaging certain areas of the foot can affect the spinal column and other parts of the body—is being practiced by some nurse-therapists. Also, meditation, stress control, and relaxation training are being taught by people with nursing degrees. Many other counseling personnel have entered some of these specialty areas, especially bio-feedback and behavioral approaches to stress control; however, I specifically mentioned nursing personnel because they are particularly good candidates due to the dual training.

Pastoral Counseling

When a person is hospitalized, it is not unusual for him to receive a visit from a clergyman. His own minister, priest, or rabbi may pay him a visit or a clergyman affiliated with the hospital may stop by. In fact, a clergyman may be the first (and only) counselor a person with a serious health problem encounters. Many clergymen have received training in human behavior and extensive counseling training, and are very qualified counselors.

A seriously ill patient may seek religious information and ask a pastoral counselor to assist him in becoming a formal member of a religious group. The patient may undergo formal training and may receive sacraments or go through other rituals. For a seriously ill person, many clergymen are happy to speed up the process. Although a person with cancer may be a member of a religious group, he may have fallen away from active participation. People with life-threatening illnesses sometimes return to active participation. A pastoral counselor can assist in that process.

Often persons struck with serious health problems believe something they did or did not do was responsible for their illness. If a patient believes he is being punished for past sins, or if he has unresolved guilt feelings, a trained pastoral counselor may be the best source of counseling. A ritual of absolution, such as follows the Catholic sacrament of confession, is a tangible washing away of the sins, and hopefully the guilt. Even a less tangible process, such as a clergyman praying or discussing the patient's feelings with him can provide considerable relief.

Rabbi Steven Moss tells the story of a woman with stomach cancer. She believed that she got that disease because she had stopped eating kosher food. She asked the Rabbi to say a prayer of repentance on her behalf. He did, and she got better. "If she didn't believe she had been excused she would have died," says the Rabbi convincingly (Moss, 1987).

Patients diagnosed with cancer very often rage at God, asking what they did to deserve this and proclaiming the good life they have led. It may be helpful to have a tangible target in the form of a symbol of God to direct that anger toward. Clergymen working in hospitals become accustomed to receiving such displaced anger. Rabbi Moss spoke to a group of cancer patients about anger and about a 19-year-old leukemia patient, named Gary, who demanded, "Where is the justice in what is happening to me?" The Rabbi could only respond, "Gary, I would be a fool if I tried to give you an answer to that." Gary asked that the Rabbi be called so he could hold his hand as he died the following day. A closeness had quickly developed because the patient perceived that the Rabbi was open and honest, and that he did not lecture about God and Fate and the Cosmos. Instead, the Rabbi came across as a vulnerable person, someone who is sometimes helpless and who doesn't pretend to have all the answers.

The Rabbi recalls another woman hitting him and screaming, "Why is your God doing this to my husband? I hate Him and I hate you." She then fell into the Rabbi's arms weeping. Later she apologized and said, "I'm sorry, I didn't mean what I said." The Rabbi said, "Yes, you did, and it's okay." Counselors should remember to affirm negative feelings when they are dealing with people who are overcome by rage and pain.

Another Jewish chaplain, Rabbi Pesach Krauss, was the first full-time

Jewish clergyman at Memorial Sloan-Kettering Cancer Center. He sees as many as 150 patients each week, patients who feel isolated and alone. Rabbi Krauss stresses the importance of touch. He operates on a feeling level. To help him understand how newly diagnosed patients feel, he recalls experiences in his own life. A trained rehabilitation counselor and family therapist, the Rabbi had a prison ministry for 15 years before beginning his work at Sloan-Kettering. He emphasizes the satisfactions that a career in pastoral counseling can bring. "The nurture I receive from the patients, the courage, the sharing of intimate feelings, the realization of the fragility of life, brings into focus my everyday blessings and clarifies my own priorities" (**Newsday**, 2 March 1986).

Support of Family and Friends

A frequent theme throughout this book has been, and will continue to be, the importance of a strong support system. In discussing the types of counseling needs in this section, it seems appropriate to again stress the on-going support and verbal encouragement of relatives and close friends. Such verbal support can be termed counseling in only the loosest sense of the word, but I believe that it fits in the continuum of verbal support and information that is helpful in dealing with cancer.

Some of the biggest advantages of the close friend, spouse, child, as a counselor are (1) it's free, (2) it's continual over a period of time, from the first fears of pre-diagnosis through recovery or death, and (3) it's accompanied most often by much genuine feeling and real personal caring. Disadvantages are chiefly that the care-giver (1) lacks objectivity, (2) can cause harmful reactions by presenting an overly positive or negative picture, or by giving incorrect or distorted information, and (3) probably lacks the counseling skills to know how best to deal with many of the patient's emotional reactions.

In addition to serving as good, concerned listeners, families and friends can help the patient in practical ways, such as making arrangements and shopping for food, clothing, medical supplies, and reading materials, including good information about the illness and how to cope with it. Family and friends can also be helpful in arranging professional help, including making appointments with medical specialists for consultation and with surgeons for second opinions, and with professional social service agencies and counselors.

Peer Counseling

Peer counseling is defined as counseling "from persons who have come to terms with their own disabilities and are able to lend support and serve as role models for others seeking to function independently" (New York University/Human Resources Center, 1983).

The value of patients helping patients has been known for some time. People who have been through the trauma of a life-threatening illness often have the desire to help others who are going through the same trauma. Cancer patients, in my talks with them, have often expressed the sentiment that there are certain things only another cancer patient can understand. That observation is probably not true. However, many patients firmly believe it. They open up more easily to another patient and share personal information more readily.

There is also the perception that the cancer survivor counsels because of an altruistic and genuine feeling for persons with cancer, that no business or scientific motive is involved. Again, the patient may be wrong about these assumptions, but he believes them nonetheless. The cancer patient has, of course, shared many similar experiences—the fear; the waiting; the uncertainty; the pain; the same, or similar, treatments. A knowing word, a quickly grasped intention, rapidly establishes a bond between two persons with cancer experiences. A social worker, visiting a patient in the hospital, may need to work much harder to establish a rapport with the patient. Of course, this is not always true. A patient may have very high regard for education and training and may be so credentials-oriented that he refuses to speak with a peer counselor, assuming that while the person may be well-meaning, he or she is unqualified and therefore not really able to help.

Like family and friends, peer counselors are usually free. The advice, support, and counsel they offer is done as a service, many say in repayment of the debt they feel as cancer survivors. They usually are affiliated with an organization and receive some training and materials from the organization. Referrals are very often provided by an organization such as a local chapter of the American Cancer Society or a local self-help group that is operated by patients.

The American Cancer Society sponsors several programs where patients help other patients. In the **CanSurmount** program, trained volunteers who have successfully coped with cancer offer support to patients. Most **CanSurmount** chapters offer services such as hospital and home visitation, and telephone peer counseling. It is designed basically as a patient visitor program; volunteers make themselves available to family members as well as patients. Some chapters of the American Cancer Society have attempted to pair patients by such factors as type and site of cancer, sex and age. The number of volunteers in some areas does not always make it possible to match peers closely, but every attempt is made to select a cancer survivor who the new patient will feel at ease with since this will facilitate communication. All cancer sites are represented in this program.

Some peer support programs are more specifically geared for certain types of cancer patients. For example, **New Voice Clubs** are organized by some ACS chapters for laryngectomees and their families and friends. Persons who have had vocal chord surgery can meet and communicate with each other at groups whimsically called **The Lost Chords.** Mastectomy groups are available in virtually all ACS Divisions; these gatherings tend to be large and well-attended. In **Reach to Recovery,** trained women who have coped successfully with mastectomy surgery, visit women before and after surgery, both in the hospital and at home. They demonstrate exercises and prostheses and offer emotional support. Patients with stomas also have their own specialized Colostomy and Ileostomy groups, organized by some ACS chapters. **Candlelighters** are groups for parents of children with cancer.

There are many patient support groups unrelated to the American Cancer Society. Some of them are sponsored by hospitals, some by churches, and some by private self-help organizations. To give the reader an idea of the range of such groups, a partial listing follows. Not all these groups have chapters throughout the country; some are regional, others local.

CHART 2

Self-Help Organizations

Compassionate Friends
A self-help group for bereaved parents.

D.E.S. Action
Self-help for women, sons, and daughters who have been exposed to D.E.S.

H.A.L.O.
Organization for patients with Hodgkin's and Lymphoma diseases.

Make Today Count
A national self-help group founded by Orville Kelly for anyone with a life-threatening disease.

Coping With Cancer
Group support for all patients and their families.

Living With Cancer
Group with guest speakers and discussion.

Andrea Hope Olicker Memorial Foundation
Group for young cancer patients, age 16 to 36 years.

Cancer Care, Inc., Groups
Various groups for cancer patients, their families, and bereaved persons.

S.H.A.R.E.
Self Help Action and Rap Experiences for post-mastectomy women and anyone with, or concerned about, breast disease.

C.H.U.M.S.
Cancer Hopefuls United for Mutual Support. A national group that sponsors group counseling sessions, educational meetings, and other services.

I Can Cope Mutual Support Group
I Can Cope is an educational program for cancer patients and their families; this group extends the experience to longer term support.

We Can Do
A cancer support based in Arcadia, California, founded by Barbara Coleman.

American Chronic Pain Association
Founded by Penney Cowan, ACPA focuses on getting people out of the patient role. Based in Monroeville, Pennsylvania.

National Chronic Pain Outreach
Started 10 years ago by Gwendolyn Talbot, this network has groups in 24 states devoted to helping people in pain regain control of their lives.

National Hospice Organization
There are more than 800 hospices around the country. Heavy reliance on volunteers lowers costs and demystifies the experience of dying.

Caring, Inc.
    Support group that includes all sites, and encourages participation of family members. Based in Manhasset, New York.

Exceptional Cancer Patients (ECaP)
    Founded in California by noted author Bernie Siegel, ECap is a specialized support group that aims for personal change and healing.

Three patient self help groups have been selected to examine in greater detail. They are **Make Today Count, We Can Do** and **CHUMS**.

Make Today Count

In 1973, a newspaperman in Iowa, Orville Kelly, learned he had cancer and felt a terrible sense of fear and isolation. He founded a support organization for those dealing with cancer or any life threatening illness which has continued through today. Kelly's challenge to cancer patients was, "Let's face it . . . and talk about it." Make Today Count, began in Burlington, Iowa but soon developed into an international organization. Patients meet in informal groups and share feelings. That is the essence of the organization. They learn sometimes to cope with the emotional trauma of illness, and of ways to appreciate their daily lives. Kelly regarded the latter point as critical. He hoped that the meetings would not develop into exercises in self-pity but rather serve as a gateway back into the mainstream of life for those whose lives were shattered by illness. Despite the positive objectives, the organization does recognize that cancer changes lives as well as relationships, and it is important to deal with these changes. The stated goals of Make Today Count are to:

• promote openness and honesty in discussing and dealing with a life threatening illness
• help the patient and family cope with the illness by providing a place where they can share their feelings and concern
• improve the quality of life for all persons with serious illness by making the community aware of the needs of the seriously ill
• assist the professional in communication with patients and families, and better meeting their emotional needs
• share in making each day count for something worthwhile and special

Orville Kelly has written much about his philosophy and ways that he believed can help people to make each day count. The following is from his book *Until Tomorrow Comes:*

• If you have needs, let them be known. No one can anticipate your needs or communicate with you effectively if you remain silent. Do not be afraid to accept help. We all need help at some time during our lives.

• You must remember that cancer is many different diseases and some types are more deadly and devastating than others. Therefore, you must not assume that a diagnosis of cancer necessarily means an early and painful death. Ask your physician what type of cancer you have. It is YOUR Cancer, and it is a violation of your rights if you are not told the truth when you seek it.

• You must also realize that with proper and effective medical treatment, you may have years of life left to you, or you may even be cured.

• Do not try to find someone to blame for your cancer. It is not your fault, your doctor's fault, or the fault of your family. Nor did God, I believe, cause your cancer. I believe cancer is God's enemy, too, and He is on my side. Realize that many people have learned to live despite this disease, with limitations, and that from suffering can come accomplishments.

• If you expect honesty from others, be honest with them and with yourself.

• Realize that hope can be kept alive through your attitude, your faith, and proper medical treatment.

• Realize, if you have a family, that your loved ones have their own unique problems with which to cope. If you turn your anger against them, it makes it terribly difficult for them to support you or to face their problems.

• If you are a cancer patient living alone, realize your problems are different from those of someone with a family. But there are things you can do to ease your loneliness. Seek out self-help groups and become involved in their work. Helping others is an effective therapy for loneliness.

• Friends may shun you, not because they don't care about you, but because they don't know what to do or say. They are afraid they might upset you or your family by saying the wrong thing. You can help to put them at ease by letting them know how you feel.

• Let your doctor know of any changes in your health or of any new pains. On the other hand, don't automatically associate every new pain or discomfort with cancer. Something else may be causing your problems.

- If you are being treated for cancer and the prognosis seems good, don't become obsessed with death. Your chance for long-term survival may be greater than some of the people who are worrying about YOU.
- It does little good to ask, "Why me?" You will get no answers.
- Do accept that lengthy depression is inevitable. It can be a tolerable emotion, unless it becomes overwhelming. But learn to find ways to ease your depression. Find reasons to live. Discover new pleasures. Many cancer patients find a release for their feelings in writing poetry or books, or in music or painting. Others discover that helping people is a very effective therapy.
- Let your doctors know you want to be a part of your own treatment. Tell them you want to cooperate with them and to have a part in you own destiny. After all, it is YOUR cancer and YOUR life.
- Consider whether or not you are REALLY protecting your loved ones if you decide to be brave and pretend "everything is all right" when it isn't. Chances are, your spouse can cope better with the truth than with deceit and "game-playing." Be honest with your children, too, because they cannot respond to your need for understanding if they are not aware of your disease and the prognosis.
- Communicate with persons around you. If some of your friends cannot accept your cancer, find new friends. But give persons a chance to accept what has happened to you.
- Consider some of the practical problems resulting from a serious illness. No one, except God, really knows when you will die. However, certain arrangements for your funeral can be made, and a will can be drawn up through your attorney. Check your insurance policies and the beneficiaries you have listed. When these things have been done, you can go on with the business of living.
- Learn about the different resources available in your community. Find out about visiting nurses, where to get help for gas to out-of-town treatments, and check to see if there is a physician in your area who will accept you as a patient.
- False hope can come in many forms. Consider the financial costs of unproven methods for treating cancer. Some unorthodox treatments sound appealing but are often costly and ineffective.
- If things are going well for you and then something goes wrong, do not panic. A relapse may not signal the end at all. Give your physicians a chance to employ their skills and the latest treatments for cancer at their disposal.
- Realize that there are diseases other than cancer that can be treated but not cured. Hypertension is one; diabetes is another.
- If you do not want pity, do not ask for it.
- If you are one who feels God will cure you if you believe strongly enough and pray long enough, know that faith and prayer are extremely important; but do not turn away from God when things do not go well.

Do not feel you are being punished by God because you have not been a good person. Once, I blamed God for my cancer, but when I turned to Him for help when I had reached bottom, I discovered that from despair and suffering can come new dreams and a new life. Do not seek success and happiness so eagerly and intently; relax, reach out to others; TRULY be a good person; and, perhaps, happiness will find YOU!

• If you do not want extraordinary measures used to keep you alive unnecessarily (when there is no hope for reasonable life), then let your family, pastor, and physicians know how you feel. At least they can consider your feelings if they must make a decision in the future.

• Do not try to hide your illness. Cancer is a disease, not a form of punishment.

• Sooner or later you will probably encounter persons who feel that cancer might be contagious. It is these persons who have problems, not you. Their fear of cancer overrides their common sense.

• Realize the importance of love. Those who love you need to express this love and you need to tell others how much you love them. Do not wait until tomorrow.

• If you consider the quality of your life and make each day count in the same way, you have just as long to live as anyone else—the rest of your life.

• Remember, you are not alone; there are others who care about you. (Kelly, 1979)

Orville Kelly lived with his cancer until his death in June 1980. He spent the final seven years of his life writing, traveling and spreading the word of the Make Today Count organization. The MTC organization is now located in Osage, Beach, Missouri. Wanda Kelly, Orville's widow, has continued to be active and involved in its future.

This writer first learned of MTC through a Cancer Information Service at Memorial Sloan-Kettering Hospital in New York City. Recovering from cancer surgery in 1980, I was seeking a support group and was referred to a Make Today Count Chapter which met every other week in lower Manhattan. There, I had the great fortune of meeting Pastor Robert Bauers, a Lutheran minister and trained social worker and psychotherapist who served as group leader. I attended Make Today Count meetings for more than two years and had the opportunity to receive and give comfort and understanding. The leader, Bob, ran the group informally and there were few rules or procedures. Postcards, reminding members of meetings, were sent out and beyond that there was little feeling of a formal organization. No officers, no speakers, no refreshments, no dues or fees, no obligations to attend or excuses for not attending. Some evenings 8 persons might show up, others only 1. Meetings were rarely cancelled. Bob ran them informally; people generally just started talking. He would sometimes offer advice or guidance, but most evenings he said little. The group was certainly not limited to talking about Orville Kelly's philosophy. In fact, one evening I recall we discussed the Simontons' work on visual imagery, and Bob led a guided imagery session. Meetings lasted from 8–10 PM. They were good for me, and then I found I no longer needed them. The benefits of the support group no longer outweighed the long wait after work in Manhattan for the group to begin and the late trek home to Long Island. This may seem a trivial aside but it illustrates an important stage that many cancer patients report— outgrowing the need to talk about the illness and the feelings connected with it. Support groups providing a safe, comfortable place for cancer patients to air their anger, frustrations, fear and hopes for the future are an important, even crucial resource, for many persons. Then, in my own experience, I woke up one morning and found I was talked out. I had expressed every conscious feeling and obtained all the information and reassurances I required. I continued for quite a while after reaching that point, primarily to offer support and a listening ear to newer members.

I have heard MTC criticized as a death-oriented organization. That was not my experience. Our chapter which met in Greenwich Village, New York, was not morbid in outlook or discussion. I recall each of the participants warmly; as a group we were hopeful and upbeat. Our chapter could have been criticized as a bit loose in format and organization perhaps. The structure and content were very casual; too casual for some people I suppose. But I found the lack of rules, expectations and rigid format just what I needed at this stressful time in my life. The emphasis was on talk and sharing and it seemed to serve the needs of many, and serve them well.

Recently, I attended a cancer patient education conference on Long Island. The group was captivated by a music therapist named Deanna Edwards, who gave an inspiring presentation in words and song called, "Music, Laughter and Tears." Ms. Edwards recalled her long friendship with Orville Kelly and gave us a sense of the mission this man felt. Make Today Count became an obsession and the culminating experience and contribution of his life. Ms. Edwards spoke of the concept of "creative grief," pointing out how a grief stricken father whose son was kidnapped and killed started a national organization to benefit missing children; how film actor Paul Newman began an organization to help critically ill children after losing his young son; and how Orville Kelly in establishing the Make Today Count organization proved again how creativity can come out of grief. Deanna Edwards told the conferees how when Orville Kelly was dying she went to say goodby and sing to him. Kelly loved it and asked her to wait a moment so he could call in a boy of 16 years who was in a room across the hallway and was suffering from leukemia. "He needs to hear you," and then Kelly asked that another person down the hall who he thought would enjoy the music be sent for, and so on, until the small hospital room was overcrowded with patients. Deanna Edwards sang and Orville Kelly died later that day. Wouldn't it be nice to do something nice for someone else on the day you die, as Orville Kelly did? (Edwards, 1987.)

We Can Do!

In the summer of 1981, I had become quite active in seeking information on various cancer support groups. The *Living With Cancer Newsletter* contained much information about activities and groups that had been formed to benefit cancer patients. In this way, I learned about a group in California, called We Can Do! I was sent a brochure which described the beginnings and activities of the group. A cancer patient, Barbara Coleman, movingly tells her personal story which culminated in 1980 with her remarkable victory over 2 brain tumors, and the forming of We Can Do! She became President, and the well known editor of the *Saturday Review,* Norman Cousins, became Chairman of the Board. In Cousins's best seller, *Anatomy of an Illness,* he tells of his victory over collagen disease, which is an arthritis-like, degenerative illness of the connective tissue which was eating away at his spine. Cousins was told that his condition was progressive and incurable. He "treated" the disease with vitamin C and laughter which he found easy to bring on by watching old comedy films.

Mrs. Coleman and Norman Cousins both believed that the contribution of the patient to his own recovery is immeasurable. They assert that the brain produces many secretions essential to combat disease and having confidence in one's ability to meet challenges helps to stimulate those lifesaving secretions. Moreover, they felt that having people who "have been through the long tunnel" could provide light for those still inside (Estes, 1980).

We Can Do! strives to help survivors increase confidence in their ability to take charge of their lives. An attempt is made for patients to assist each other in better understanding the quality of life. "We bolster one another and mobilize our strength to fight for life. We learn to face alienation, mutilation, fear and mortality. We learn to cope when we are faced with the staggering blow of a recurrence. We give hope without compromising realistic expectations" (**We Can Do!**, 1981).

It seems to Barbara Coleman that there is no medicine as potent as the human spirit. We Can Do! strives to nourish that spirit and keep it receptive to the positive attitudes of healing and wellness. The aim of We Can Do! simply stated is to remove fear, anger, guilt, resentment, self-condemnation and powerlessness. Some of the tenets of the We Can Do! philosophy involve growing in the acceptance of life and the helping experience:

1. Awe of life—of the whole, of the power that is put into our hands.

2. Acceptance of death—and of the inevitability of mistakes; of the new areas we have not faced; of the courage to try and fail and be willing to try again.

3. Awe of individuality—of each person and yet understanding the sameness of humankind (We Can Do!, 1981)

Barbara Coleman spells out the philosophy of her organization further in a descriptive brochure. She also explains the activities available at the weekly support meetings.

We Can Do! extends beyond medicine—we offer our cancer sufferers encouragement, love, friendship, and weekly support. We offer our services for the family members also.

We Can Do! is based totally on the acceptance of each other and where we are right now. There is no judgement, only acceptance. We are in the support group to help one another through the problem areas of disease (dis-ease). We use music, laughter, relaxation, visualization, and—most important—a positive attitude, "I am getting better and better with each day."

We think of ourselves in different stages of wellness—we do not "feel" sick; we feel only a different degree of wellness. We have a definite belief in our own recovery. As we work with our physicians, our support group, and by taking charge of our own treatment, we begin to feel better.

When we let go of fear, we do have peace of mind.

We Can Do! offers educational material at each session, incorporating the teachings of Buber, Jung, Neumann, Kierkegaard, Tillish, Berdyaev, and Teilhard de Chardin. We feel this material gives each of us an opportunity to broaden our perspective on life. It also, in a real sense, gives us something to think about other than our disease.

We have a real learning and sharing experience each week. This experience is then carried out during the following week by our tele- phone network—offering our experiences to those who may not have been at the past session. We keep in touch constantly.

No one is alone.

The pilot group of We Can Do! consisted of fifty-one survivors, six family members, the director and three professionals, including two clinical psychologists.

Each week we add new survivors and family members. As the group increases, we divide into smaller groups of 10 or 12, each with a clinical psychologist and the director of the project supervising.

Group Process

Music is an important part of each weekly session. We begin each meeting with at least 15 minutes of music as the people arrive.

Music therapy seems to be important to relaxation and allows the group to mingle.

After the music, we begin each session seated in a circle. We request a positive thought from everyone present at this time.

We feel that by expressing some positive thing that has occurred during the past week, it seems to free the mind of negativity.

Each member feels a responsibility to not let the next person down; therefore, he will have some positive statement to make.

It is very important that there be no pressure applied to induce a positive response because sometimes a member really has not had a very positive week and he must be able to feel guilt-free if he does not respond—in other words—no pressure on any member.

We are finding that laughter seems to help with the healing process— not forced jokes—sometimes a humorous situation involving a member or his family, a favorite story perhaps—anything that induces real laughter. Each week, more and more members are finding some humor in their lives.

Visualization

The key to valid visualization is realizing that the process is not logical. Example: tiny fish in the blood stream eating cancer cells, spitting them out and "seeing" the dead cells being eliminated through natural channels, then "seeing" them as they are flushed down the toilet—not logical, but it works!!

Some group members have found it difficult to visualize. With the help of others, we seem to come up with an appropriate visualization for that particular member.

After a few weeks, we have found that we know one another well enough to support each other in visualization as well as in other areas.

We Can Do! members feel that visualization is one of the key tools to be used in their recovery!

Learning Process

Before we begin our learning process each week, we find it to be helpful for the members to share and discuss mainly their feelings, chemotherapy and anything that is particularly positive or negative that they may need help with in this day.

Then we begin with almost a classroom instruction period where we introduce new thought patterns, new ways to help modify a life style, methods to activate human capabilities and some psychological methods that help one deal with one's unique state of being. We are helping members dissolve barriers that prevent optimum health.

We introduce the philosophers, the positive psychologists of our time and try to give each member a workable plan for the coming week.

After the learning process, we come together for a period of relaxation.

Relaxation

We use Carl Simonton's relaxation techniques.

We Can Do! has also developed some of its own tapes.

The relaxation is approximately a 15-minute process.

It is important to come out of this process slowly. We repeat "I am getting better and better with each day" three times quietly or to ourselves.

We embrace one another with love and friendship which will sustain us until out next session.

(We Can Do!, 1981).

I wrote to Mrs. Coleman in August 1981, since I had learned of a study that We Can Do! was conducting of cancer survivors. It involved completing a questionnaire based on Jung's theory of types. The idea of the study was to examine differences in effectiveness of various types of self-healing techniques e.g. visualization, affirmation, realization, for different personality types. An extended discussion of self-healing methods and techniques will appear later in this book.

Chums

Since becoming a cancer survivor I affiliated with several patient self-help groups, but the group that I became most involved with was CHUMS. The acronym stands for Cancer Hopefuls United for Mutual Support. CHUMS was founded by a very dynamic lady who I came to know quite well, Sarah Splaver. A colleague clipped an article about CHUMS from the *New York Times.* Dr. Splaver, a psychologist, was interviewed by the *Times.* She pointed out that although statistics indicate that there are several million people with a history of cancer alive, one doesn't seem to run into very many. Most are afraid to say they had cancer. Dr. Splaver discussed the organization she has founded and the many services it provides. These include discussion sessions among patients, educational meetings and phone-a-patient, and visit-a-patient programs. The organization sounded interesting to me since it involved more than just patient discussion sessions. As valuable a service as that is and as much as I has benefited from it earlier, I had outgrown a need for it by this point. I was, however, intrigued with the more activist activities implied in the *Times* article. Mention was made, for example, of lobbying to outlaw job discrimination against people who have had cancer. I was ready for a group like this.

Over the next few years, I became increasingly more involved in CHUMS and served on the Board of Directors for 2 years. Among those who lent their names as honorary Trustees of CHUMS were Marilyn Cooper, Tony award winning actress; Geraldine Ferraro, Congresswoman and Vice Presidential Candidate, Candy Jones, Talk Show Host and Author; Barbara Mikulski, Congresswoman and Daniel P. Moynihan, U.S. Senator.

The CHUMS brochure describes the organization as a national coalition of cancer patients, survivors and their families and friends. The stated purposes of CHUMS follow:

1. To offer therapeutic aid via self-help and crisis intervention.
2. To afford cancer patients/survivors the opportunity to share experiences, and offer each other mutual peer support.
3. To help cancer patients/survivors and their families and friends all the better to cope with and reduce the resulting traumas and problems of cancer.

4. To disseminate information about the latest developments on the subject of cancer (inclusive of lecture-discussions by prominent cancer specialists).

5. To stress that cancer is a disease, not a disaster, and that it often is curable, especially if detected early and treated early.

6. To counter misconceptions that cancer is a "death sentence" by highlighting cancer survivors who are five and more years beyond diagnosis.

7. To encourage cancer patients to become cancer "hopefuls" and opt for life.

8. To improve the quality of life of cancer patients/survivors by helping them to strengthen their "psychological weapons" positive outlook, cheerful attitude, hope, optimism, the determination to live, and the will to get well, be well and stay well.

Dr. Splaver published an ambitious agenda.

1. Crisis Intervention and Information Service on a nationwide basis.

2. Self-help Rap Sessions at which cancer patients/survivors share experiences with each other.

3. Educational meetings at which prominent cancer specialists speak and answer questions.

4. Phone-a-Patient and Visit-a-Patient Programs to let cancer patients know somebody cares.

5. Parties and get-togethers for everyone's enjoyment.

6. Campaign against discrimination of cancer patients/survivors in employment, financial, insurance, and other areas.

7. Stimulate research in the fields of virology and immunology where, we believe, a cure for cancer will be found.

8. CHUMS EXCHANGE, a newsletter with good news for and about cancer patients/survivors.

I personally attended many lectures sponsored by CHUMS and found them all highly informative. I met a number of remarkable cancer survivors through the organization, a few of whom I still occasionally hear from. Sarah Splaver is a person of great energy and she is the highest form of optimist. She has devoted countless hours to the organization and gave cancer survivors much hope since her optimism is so infectious. She was able to attract quite a bit of publicity for her cause and for a more positive image of cancer patients and survivors. She lashes out at the "death-myth" which promotes the idea that everyone who gets cancer will die. Dr. Splaver has pointed out the prevalence of that negative image in films, books and the media, and strives to challenge it.

Sarah Splaver has left the active direction of CHUMS and has moved to Florida. Although I have not had recent direct involvement with the organization, I've heard that a less ambitious organization continues and regular meetings are held at Lenox Hill Hospital in New York City.

Examination of those three self-help groups illustrates the range and variety of philosophies and activities. CHUMS proposes perhaps the broadest and most ambitious agenda, but in my experience much of that agenda was left undone. When an organization needs to rely on volunteer help, objectives must be modest. The objectives of CHUMS have sometimes been not only grand but grandiose. Much time and money is needed to fulfill such a program. Providing salaries or any type of remuneration for the workers in self-help groups is often difficult if not impossible. Dues, fund raising events, raffles, luncheons, etc., are not enough to provide an on-going salary for a Director. Devoting energy to raising money for the organization can defeat the purpose of a self-help group, and disillusion the members.

In some ways Make Today Count seems not to stretch its wings wide enough. But perhaps keeping to a simple, do-able goal of providing support discussions among patients is a wise course of action.

Professionals sometimes belittle the overly-enthusiastic language one often finds in materials published by self-help groups. There tends to be a combination of 1960s "love philosophy" and enthusiastic, touchy-feely proselytizing in some of the brochures and literature printed. A subjective and optimistic philosophy is harmless and excusable, I think, when the motivation is pure and the results are positive.

Professional Counselors As Group Leaders

In addition to support groups that are led or facilitated by peers— persons with a cancer history—several organizations sponsor group counseling sessions led by professionally trained personnel. Peer leaders may have some training, but it is usually minimal, often consisting of several sessions totaling 8 to 12 hours. Courses may cover resources in the community, medical aspects of cancer treatment and management, emotional reactions to having cancer, and the rudiments of counseling principles. Formal university level training in a helping profession is ordinarily not required.

When the task is to assist a group of persons with cancer in a group counseling setting, it is debatable whether the "real life" cancer experience is as valuable or even more so, than is a formal advanced education in a helping profession. There has been little documentation of the value of support groups of any type.

A **Reach to Recovery** program was evaluated in the Boston area. A total of 90 women who had undergone breast surgery were divided into three groups. One group received no program visitors; another group was visited by peer volunteers from **Reach to Recovery**; the third group was visited by a person trained in interpersonal communication skills. The mastectomy patients reported 1 to 3 months later that all visitors—whether volunteers or someone who had been trained—were helpful. The group that had been visited by the trained person was judged to be functioning better, however. The author of the study, Ms Linda Brown, reported that less expression of anger, less dependence on tranquilizing medication, and less use of alcohol was manifest by women in the third group; this led her to conclude that the women who were visited by an especially trained person at the time of their surgery profited the most (Krant, 1978).

Many workers have indicated that there is a need for further evaluation of the effectiveness of support groups, both those with untrained peer leaders and those led by persons with formal counseling training.

Professionally led groups may be found throughout the country. In San Francisco, for example, several groups were formed at Mt. Zion Hospital. One group consisted of young patients, while a second group contained older patients. A third group was formed for family members. All three groups were led by a trained social worker or a psychologist, and a psychiatrist was available for back-up assistance. Federal funds supported this project, which is reportedly no longer active (Krant, 1978).

The literature also contains reports of a multi-family therapy group in Los Angeles that is directed by a clinical psychologist. A program called **At Home Rehabilitation Project,** which operates out of the Cancer Center, Inc., in Cleveland, Ohio, offers a home rehabilitation team. A social worker serves as a team coordinator, but a public health nurse, a physical therapist, an occupational therapist, a child life worker, a vocational-educational counselor, and a health educator are also on staff. The program's brochure notes that "experienced counseling to help you and your family adjust to the impact of illness. Will arrange for other supportive services and consultants as needed." The brochure also notes that the program is supported by a contract from the National Cancer Institute.

A New York newspaper reports that in Long Island, N.Y., the **Adelphi University School of Social Work** offers counseling for individuals, couples, families, and groups.

Cancer Care is another organization that offers individual and group counseling. It is led by professionally trained human service personnel, usually social workers.

Despite the number of lay and professional counseling resources available, both fee-charging and free, some persons with cancer do not seem to avail themselves of any form of personal counseling assistance. In some parts of the country, some of the resources that have been mentioned may not be available. Many people are not amenable to asking for, or receiving, counseling help. However, one form of assistance is available, and although it is not quite counseling in a formal sense, it can impart information and comfort. That resource is the printed word. Counseling by leaflet, books, and pamphlets is perhaps the widest and most common form of assistance sought by cancer patients. The American Cancer Society, as well as other teaching and voluntary organizations, sends out thousands of booklets to patients and family members yearly. The titles of several booklets are listed below:

Are You or Your Loved One a Cancer Patient? published by Can Surmount, ACS.

You Are Not Alone, published by ACS.

When a Family Faces Cancer, by Elizabeth Ogg, Public Affairs Pamphlet no. 286, published by the Public Affairs Committee, New York, N.Y.

Taking Time, published by the U.S. Dept of Health and Human Services, Washington, D.C.

Help Yourself — Tips for Teenagers with Cancer, published by Adria Laboratories and NCI.

The Dying Person and the Family, by Nancy Doyle, Public Affairs Pamphlet no. 485, published by the Public Affairs Committee, New York, N.Y.

This list is by no means complete, but it does present a picture of the variety and range of areas booklets cover. All of these publications are either free or available at a nominal cost.

Many persons who would not even consider seeing a counselor will read a booklet and perhaps get some valuable information or needed comfort.

Hot Lines are another form of "counseling," although not in the truest sense. Many large cancer centers, universities, and voluntary organizations operate telephone information services. They are sometimes limited to specific areas, such as Adelphi University's telephone service for women with breast cancer. Some are extremely comprehensive. The Cancer Information Service, for example, (1-800-4-CANCER) provides up-to-date materials about cancer to both patients and professionals. The yellow pages of phone books in most large cities provide several cancer referral and/or information services.

Other Forms of Patients Helping Patients

In recent years the rehabilitation field has broadened its constituency to include newly disabled persons, and people who are often more severely disabled. Traditional rehabilitation programs that are vocationally oriented have been supplemented by programs with a different goal—stressing independent living for persons with handicapping conditions.

The Rehabilitation Act of 1973 made possible a new concept in rehabilitating disabled people by establishing independent living programs. The aim is for persons with all types of handicaps to become productive members of mainstream society, relying less on family and friends. Independent living centers have been set up throughout the country to help disabled persons move toward this goal. A basic tenet of these centers is that everyone has the right to make basic decisions regarding his or her lifestyle. Services vary from center to center, but generally they include counseling, referrals for attendant care, advocacy services concerning legal and economic rights and benefits, housing and transportation assistance, and training in seeking job skills. Most of the services are free.

The basic requirement for persons residing in independent living centers is that they be severely handicapped by a physical or mental disability, and in need of one or more services offered by the center so they can live more independently or can secure and keep jobs. Although many persons with cancer qualify under this definition, relatively few take advantage of this resource.

The families of cancer patients often do not know where to go for advice or how to obtain medical equipment or to get legal counseling or to arrange for transportation. The recovering cancer patient may find counseling groups whose members are learning to live with physical limitations. The center may also help those who are trying to reenter the labor market (Conti, 1982). Persons with cancer seeking independent living centers in their communities should call or write to their State Vocational Rehabilitation Program, which is listed in the telephone book under State Services, and should inquire about the nearest Independent Living Center.

Peer counseling is a service commonly offered by independent living centers. Moses, Barell, and Siler (1982) have defined a peer counselor as "a disabled person who has disability-related experiences, knowledge and coping skills, and assists other disabled individuals with their disability-related experiences."

Some feel that peer counselors may be uniquely able to understand and interact with consumers. Some peer counselors focus on teaching independent living skills, others emphasize psychological counseling, while still others concentrate on sharing community resources (Pittman and Mathews, 1984).

In discussing the growth of self-help groups for cancer patients, Cox (1975) asserts that the patient must be an integral part of planning and determining what other patients need—in terms of information and supportive services. He sees the cancer patient as an educator and a counselor, and during a 3-year project at the Mayo Comprehensive Cancer Center, Cox strived to promote and stretch that role. Her book, *Living with Lung Cancer* (1977), was edited cover to cover by patients. She believes that patients with cancer are helped in their adjustment to the disease, and even to their impending death, by being allowed to help other patients. In the Mayo program, cancer patients helped develop printed materials and audio visual materials, as well as counseling programs and psychological support programs.

Some cancer survivors become strong advocates for patient rights after going through traumatic experiences as a patient. A good example is Caroline Sperling, whose story was told in the *Washington Post* in 1984. Ms. Sperling was a terminal cancer patient in 1979, having experienced a recurrence of breast cancer with a metastasis into her abdomen. She was given six months to two years to live. She actively fought the disease, using the Simonton imagery techniques and consciously took responsibility for her treatment program. She considered various medical options and selected the one she felt right about—a lumpectomy. She also entered an extensive psychotherapy program. She believes that this approach eliminated all signs of active cancer in her body. Ms. Sperling, who now counsels cancer patients and their families at the **Cancer Counseling Institute,** a service she established in her home in Bethesda, Maryland, is president of the International Association of Cancer Counselors. She strongly believes that cancer is a warning that something has gone wrong with a person's life, and that it can lead to a special time of learning when mistaken attitudes and maladaptive patterns can be changed and a new life begun.

In 1978, Richard A. Block had virtually retired from his business, the H&R Block tax preparation chain, to relax and enjoy his success. He was diagnosed with inoperable lung cancer and told that nothing could be done to save him. He aggressively sought out the best care possible; in two years he was told that his cancer was in complete remission. Mr. Block believes that other patients could also survive if they take charge of their care program, and if they have access to the most expert advice. In 1982 he told *The New York Times* that he and his wife were setting up a non-profit center to provide cancer patients with fast and up-to-date information provided by a panel of top cancer experts. The first **R.A. Block Cancer Management Center** was opened in Kansas City. Several other centers have since opened around the country. Like many cancer patients, Mr. Block vowed to spend the rest of his life helping others hit with cancer, and he appears to have the determination, the integrity, and the financial resources to stick to his promise.

In addition to survival and medical management, cancer survivors are left with many other concerns. A Detroit man, Paul Boyd, developed cancer of the spine in 1980 at the age of 29 years. Radiation treatments eliminated the tumor but damaged spinal cord nerve endings, leaving Boyd paralyzed from the waist down and confined to a wheelchair. First he lost his job. Then his marriage ended. Life looked unpromising. Although depressed, he forced himself to participate in an intensive exercise program, strapping himself onto a stationary bike and peddling 1700 miles over the next two years. He was able to leave the wheelchair for crutches, and then left the crutches for a walker; now he can walk slowly with the assistance of a cane. His cancer is in remission, and he has thrown himself into a new mission with fervor: helping persons with handicaps find friendship, and maybe even love. Boyd has started a dating service for the physically challenged called **Special People**. Newspaper reports indicate a good deal of interest in the service, which is seen by many as a major, yet unmet, need for persons with disabilities (Biggs, 1985).

With the proliferation of self-help groups and patient-helping-patient volunteer programs, the importance of guidance and training for volun-

CHART 3

Qualities of a Volunteer

A Good Volunteer	A Bad Volunteer
Shows his/her interest by her own attitude in mind, countenance, and body language	Appears bored or disinterested, hurried or impersonal
Provides quiet assurance, draws other person out	Dominates, imposes opinions, forces dependency
Encourages, is patient, optimistic	Is critical of hospital or doctors, is pessimistic
Demonstrates sensitivity to the individual	Fails to empathize, is set on delivering literature and keeping to a format
Displays a sense of humor, appropriately	Has no humor—deadpan (morbid)
Realizes that to serve as a volunteer is to let the other people rise and shine	Takes advantage of his/her role to discuss his/her own medical history and background
Checks with nursing staff	Comes and goes, unrecognized
Allows for personal space and yet not too far	Stands at foot of bed

Four Helpful Hints for a Volunteer

1. Don't interrupt. (Very dangerous with cancer patients because it is hard enough to have them talk about their diagnosis and or problems.)
2. Don't probe—below level of comfortability.
3. DON'T GIVE MEDICAL ADVICE.
4. Don't judge.

teer counselors needs to be borne in mind. In training volunteers for a local **CanSurmount** Program, the American Cancer Society offered the suggestions contained in Chart 3, "Qualities of a Volunteer."

The advice in Chart 3 might seem obvious, and even insulting, to some trained persons. It must be remembered, however, that many volunteer programs accept people with no training in human behavior and no experience in counseling. With a short orientation program, they are sent forth to work with the seriously ill, often emotionally vulnerable, people. Tips such as the one's listed above can foster confidence, and a feeling of some concrete do's and don'ts before one attempts to offer comfort and guidance for the first time.

Rehabilitation Counseling

Because of advances in the diagnosis and treatment of some cancers, there are now more than 5 million cancer survivors and 3 million 5 years past diagnosis. Some of these survivors are permanently and totally disabled. Others have some physical limitations, but with assistance they could have an improved quality of life. Still others can be helped through vocational rehabilitation services to enter or reenter the job market.

In an earlier section the Independent Living Program was discussed as one alternative for persons with cancer who were seeking to decrease their dependency and to improve their quality of life. The larger and older part of the rehabilitation field focuses on rehabilitating disabled persons into employment. The Federal/State program of vocational rehabilitation began in 1920 with the first comprehensive Vocational Rehabilitation Act, which was intended primarily for returning disabled servicemen of World War I. Since that time, the Act has been expanded to include virtually all physical and mental disabilities. Disabled persons are served through programs supported by the Rehabilitation Services Administration, an agency of the U. S. Department of Education. Applicants go to local offices, administered by the State office of vocational rehabilitation, which receives joint Federal/State funding.

The Federal/State Vocational Rehabilitation Program may provide an array of services, including (1) medical examination to determine the extent of the disability, (2) medical treatment to reduce disability, (3) counseling to determine a person's employment potential, interests, and needs, (4) training, (5) some financial help during the rehabilitation process, and (6) job placement.

Since 1965 the Vocational Rehabilitation Act has been extending its services to cancer patients. In 1978 the Independent Living Program was added. Relatively few cancer patients and survivors are served by these programs, however. It is not totally clear why this is the case.

The legality of serving clients with a history of malignancies is not a problem. The Rehabilitation Services Administration has permitted such persons to be accepted for service since 1965. Former Commissioner Robert R. Humphreys was called upon to clarify the issue 15 years later.

It is RSA's position that persons disabled by cancer **may** be eligible for vocational rehabilitation services and that such services should be provided if the individual wants to work and **can** work even if for a limited period of time. The services should be individually tailored according to the needs of the individual and the anticipated work life.

Some cancers like the lymphomas and Hodgkins Disease are similar in their outlook to multiple sclerosis. Others require extensive physical restoration services. In general, it is appropriate for vocational rehabilitation to provide job-related follow-up restorative services as needed, after primary surgical/x-ray and/or chemotherapeutic care has been provided.

Persons who are handicapped by cancer present special problems of eligibility. But over the years, a few principles have been established:
1) Persons handicapped by cancer usually have a potential for work for a significant period of time.
2) The potential for work is dependent on a number of variables, notably the natural history of the cancer involved, the individualized manner in which the specific cancer affects the patient and the personal characteristics and opportunities of the patient. [Emphasis in original]
U.S. Dept. of H.E.W., 1980.

Despite clarification and reassurance of eligibility by Federal administrators, State employed rehabilitation counselors have served far fewer persons with cancer than might be expected (U.S. Dept. of Education, 1987). Between 1971 and 1979, the number of persons with malignancies who were rehabilitated by the Federal/State Vocational Rehabilitation system increased from 1,000 to 1,556. This gain is poor considering that more than a quarter million disabled people were closed as rehabilitated in each of those years. The successful closure rate for persons with cancer in any year examined by Taylor (1981) never exceeded 0.54%.

More recent statistics are no more encouraging. In 1985, 339,688 disabled people in the VR program were closed following rehabilitation services. Of those, 218,039 were closed as successes (i.e. rehabilitations), and 121,659 persons were not rehabilitated. Of those identified as persons with cancer, 1,033 were successfully rehabilitated, and 559 were not (U.S. Dept. of Education, 1987). Simply stated, these figures indicate that one half of one percent (0.50%) of all persons rehabilitated by the vocational rehabilitation program in 1985 were clients with a cancer diagnosis.

When we look at services in general, rather than rehabilitations alone, we see that in a single recent year only 1,633 persons with cancer progressed through the VR system even as far as the planning stage (U.S. Dept. of Education, 1987). In that same year, according to the American Cancer Society, about 900,000 new cases of cancer were diagnosed (American

Cancer Society, 1987). Although survival rate estimates vary widely, we can safely predict, using the most conservative data, that between 40–50 percent of those diagnosed will survive at least five years ($\geq 385,000$).

Not all cancer survivors need, desire or qualify for VR services, of course, but those feasible for rehabilitation, and wanting VR services, are surely greater in number than the few the system has served. Analysis of the above incidence data reveals that .0018% of newly diagnosed cancer patients progressed to a planning stage in the VR system. If one were to consider the larger universe of cancer survivors, rather than just newly diagnosed cases, the percentage served by VR drops to an even smaller figure.

Although it is clear that the pool of potential workers with a cancer history has not been fully tapped by VR, the reasons for that remain somewhat of a puzzle.

Contributing factors may include hopelessness on the part of persons with cancer, and prejudice or a lack of information on the part of counselors and state administrators (Conti, 1981).

Brickner (1978) suggests three reasons why cancer patients are rarely involved in vocational rehabilitation:

(1) The lack of up-to-date information on treatment and prognosis of the disease on the part of vocational rehabilitation professionals.

(2) The lack of a comprehensive educational program on the potentials of persons whose cancer has been cured or contained; and

(3) The lack of consideration of rehabilitative goals and vocational planning early in the treatment.

Researchers have also considered that cost might be a factor. However, financial constraints probably can be discarded as a valid reason since it has been shown that the cost of closed cancer cases is the lowest per case of all compared disabilities (including tuberculosis, diabetes, mental disorders, heart disease, and orthopedic problems). Several studies have confirmed that money is not the reason. One such study found that the $370 average cost spent on a cancer client was about one third of that spent on a client with a coronary disorder. Although similar-benefit funding sources are available, they are not even being tapped (Taylor, 1984).

Perhaps cancer patients are not being made aware of the rehabilitation program. The Rehabilitation Act has had little impact on the rehabilitation of cancer patients according to a Mayo Clinic study. Employers, labor unions, and the general public, generally do not recognize that cancer survivors are able to return to work and that they are excellent candidates for vocational rehabilitation counseling. Rather than emphasizing the reality that many persons who are either cured or in a stage of cancer containment will live long, productive lives, public education programs have instead emphasized information about early warning signs of cancer, benefits of early treatment, and preventive health measures. Information on cancer and employment is particularly needed by three groups: industrial physicians, recovered cancer patients who lack adequate job skills and counselors (Brickner, 1978).

The primary reason for the underrepresentation of cancer survivors in VR, however, seems to result from the bias of the rehabilitation counselor (Taylor, 1984). Counselors' attitudes have been demonstrated to be a major obstacle to those persons receiving vocational rehabilitation services. Cancer has been shown to pose the greatest personal threat to counselors when compared with other disabilities, such as renal failure, paraplegia, and heart disease (Pinkerton and Nelson, 1978). The counselor apparently distances himself as much as possible from the cancer client, threatened by some of the same fears as those experienced by the individual with cancer. A "bad economy" or "restrictive program regulations" are commonly used excuses for not adequately serving persons with malignancies (McAleer, 1975).

The psychological, social, and vocational problems of the person with a cancer diagnosis are not so different from those of other disabled persons. Some researchers report the primary difference as the ever-present fear that the disease will progress or recur (Healey and Zislis, 1981). But fear of progression of illness is shared by many other disability groups including people with multiple sclerosis, and some forms of visual impairment, such as retinitis pigmentosa and diabetic retinopathy. Recurrence of illness also is not limited to cancer clients; persons with psychiatric disabilities, for example, have always expressed such a fear, often on sound grounds. The physical restoration problems of cancer clients require therapeutic measures similar to those provided other physically limited individuals.

In examining the most recent national statistics available on rehabilitation success, (U.S. Dept. of Education, 1987), we find that the rehabilitation rate (or success ratio) of cancer patients (63%) compares favorably with the total population of disabled individuals (64%). Since cancer is a severe disability, it is more proper to compare the rehabilitation rate with that of other severely disabled clients (62.7%). We may therefore say that cancer survivors, when given the opportunity to participate in a rehabilitation program, do about the same, or even slightly better than others with severe disabilities.

Vocational planning for the cancer client requires that the counselor consider many factors, including the part of the body involved, functional limitations, success in physical restoration, motivation, family support and psychological adjustment. Employer attitudes and the client's education and work history will all have a bearing on the formulation of a vocational plan. Chart 4, "Factors in Rehabilitation Potential Assessment for Cancer Patients," may serve as a guide in vocational planning and goal setting (Healy and Zislis, 1981).

The goals of successful employment for the cancer client requires the cooperation and coordination of many professionals. After the client's rehabilitation potential has been established, specific vocational options can be considered. Physical and environmental job demands and the client's education and work history, as well as the status of his disease, will all enter into the evaluation. The length of training programs may be affected by morbidity and life-expectancy prognosis.

Educating the community and employers is the responsibility of many persons, including rehabilitation professionals. Negative attitudes particularly those of pity, fear, and revulsion—create employment obstacles as difficult, frustrating, and unfair as any architectural barrier. Such barriers, for example, limit the employment options of clients who have had disfiguring surgery.

Chart 5, "Guide to Occupational Demands for Cancer Patients After Rehabilitation Services," describes the work demands of many occupations (Healy and Zislis, 1981).

Although the Rehabilitation Act of 1973, and its amendments, addresses many of the legislative needs of persons with a cancer history, other legislative initiatives, particularly aimed at financial help, are needed at the State level. Health insurance payments for the services of professional personnel, such as rehabilitation counselors, pastoral counselors, and other trained human service workers, is usually not reimbursable. Counseling professionals who are more widely accepted—for example, psychologists and social workers—are not accepted third-party providers in many circumstances. State legislatures need to deal with these real financial issues.

In order for rehabilitation counselors to become accepted treatment

CHART 4
Factors in Rehabilitation Potential Assessment for Cancer Patients

Positive (+)	Questionable (?)	Negative (−)
Cancer completely irradicated	Prevailing statistical information indicates that the specific cancer has a high incidence of metastasis and/or shortened life expectancy	Cancer not completely removed
No local spread		Cancer shows local spread
No evidence of distant metastasis (e.g., to other organs or bones)		Cancer shows regional lymph node spread
		Evidence of distant metastasis to organs or bones
Cancer remission by chemotherapy or radiation therapy	Duration and degree of response of the cancer to, for example, chemotherapy or radiation therapy is uncertain although some remission is noted	Cancer not responding to chemotherapy or radiation therapy
Functional losses are temporary		Functional losses are permanent
Patient is made independent through rehabilitation	Patient participating in rehabilitation program	Maximal functional independence not achieved
Good adjustment to disability		Poor adjustment to disability and not amenable to psychological counseling
Strong family support		Little or no family support

CHART 5
Guide to Occupational Demands for Cancer Patients after Rehabilitation Services
(x indicates patient usually cannot meet occupational demands)

			Musculoskeletal Amputees					Nervous System					
Occupational Demands	Breast	Head & Neck	Upper	Lower	Colo-rectal Digestive	Leukemia Lymphoma	Brain	Spinal Cord Paraplegia	Quadriplegia	Peripheral	Lung	Genito Urinary	Skin
Cosmesis		x	x										
Writing							x		x	x			
Speech		x					x						
Employer resistance		x	x				x	x	x	x			
Sedentary													
Light lifting									x	x			
Moderate lifting			x	x				x	x	x			
Heavy lifting	x	x	x	x	x	x	x	x	x	x	x	x	
Prolonged standing				x		x	x	x	x	x			
Bending, squatting, stooping				x			x	x	x	x			
Climbing				x			x	x	x	x			
High-speed performance						x	x		x	x			
Manual Skills			x				x		x	x			
Balancing skills				x			x	x	x	x			
Environmental stresses			x	x		x	x	x	x	x			
Visual-motor skills							x		x	x			
Intellectual skills							x						

Healey and Zislis, 1981

providers, the entire rehabilitation system may need to reevaluate its procedures, past efforts, and priorities with regard to persons with cancer.

There are many valuable services that rehabilitation counselors can offer, including vocational counseling, psychological counseling, crisis intervention counseling (especially at the time of diagnosis), and advice about prostheses in the cases of post-mastectomy and amputation.

The role of the rehabilitation counselor as a member of the professional cancer rehabilitation team needs to be emphasized, especially to physicians who may not be aware of, or who harbor misconceptions or prejudices about, the training and competencies of the rehabilitation counseling profession. Perhaps personal contact with competent counseling personnel is the most effective way of educating and changing misconceptions among colleagues in health, education, mental health and other related fields. It might be worthwhile for VR state directors and office managers to consider sending some knowledgeable, personable, and articulate counselors to staff meetings of local American Cancer Society chapters so they can make brief presentations about how rehabilitation counselors are trained and what their roles are. Many ACS chapters would likely welcome such in-service training because it would give many nursing, administrative, and patient services personnel the opportunity to hear for the first time about the contributions rehabilitation counselors can make.

Nor is what the field of rehabilitation counseling has to offer people with a history of cancer even universally known or accepted within the narrow area of cancer rehabilitation. A few years ago the *Journal of Rehabilitation* reported on an exemplary program in cancer rehabilitation at New York's Memorial Sloan-Kettering Hospital (McLaughlin, 1984). This writer was surprised to discover that no rehabilitation counselors were reported on the comprehensive staff. Funded by the National Cancer Institute, the project was charged with developing a model system of rehabilitation services for patients. The *Journal* article painstakingly described staff roles, especially in the fields of medicine, social work, and nutrition, but not a word is mentioned about rehabilitation counseling. This is especially surprising in a city that trains graduate level rehabilitation counselors in four universities.

A few efforts to call attention to the potential contributions of rehabilitation counselors to clients having cancer histories have been made. In the state of Virginia, an excellent *Counselor Cancer Handbook* has been developed (Franco, 1978). Commissioner Altamont Dickerson of the

Virginia Dept. of Rehabilitation Services opens the handbook with an upbeat and encouraging open letter in which rehabilitation counselors are urged to increase outreach to those persons with a diagnosis of cancer. We are informed that the handbook has been revised from time to time; updated resource listings are prepared by students and mailed to holders of the book. More such resources are needed before counselors will begin to feel comfortable working with cancer patients and survivors.

State agency administrators and rehabilitation counselors should be encouraged to learn more about this specialty area. No national conference on cancer rehabilitation has been held. No priority attention for grants aimed at rehabilitating severely disabled individuals with a history of cancer has been extended. There is no cooperative agreement between RSA and the American Cancer Society, perhaps the oldest and largest organization representing disabled consumer interests (established 1913). Steps ought to be taken to address each of these deficiencies.

The resource is called *The Challenge of Cancer Rehabilitation: A Handbook for Vocational Rehabilitation Counselors.* Many professionals contributed sections and included their perspectives on oncology, nutrition, occupational therapy, psychiatry, physical therapy, psychiatry, and happily, rehabilitation counseling. There is, in fact, a large section on Counseling and Guidance, with contributions from rehabilitation counselors, pastoral counselors, and sexual counselors. Patricia C. Franco, a rehabilitation counselor, offers a protocol, reproduced here as Chart 6, as a guideline for counseling the newly diagnosed cancer patient (Franco, 1978).

CHART 6

Psychosocial Assessment and Intervention Procedures

Time of Contact	Content of Assessment/Treatment Contact
Diagnosis or Initial Contact	**Preparation of Initial Contact** Obtain relevant information, including age, sex, marital status, living situation, finances, insurance coverage, diagnosis and procedures planned, and pre-existing medical conditions. **Initial Client Contact** A. Initiate contact to introduce self to client and explain counselor's role and Agency's policy and procedure, including. 1. Assisting client in identifying problems and potential resources and solutions.

2. Serving as liaison if needed to assist client in getting information and clarification needs.
3. Providing opportunity for expression of feelings and concerns.

B. Begin exploring with the client any current concerns he/she may wish to discuss, such as:
   1. History of onset of symptoms.
   2. Current medical situation and treatment plan.
   3. Expectation of possible changes related to tx modality; i.e., body image, impairments and pain
   4. Anticipated adjustments in functional life situations.
   5. Personal and family history, including pre-morbid behavior pattern (normal stress patterns).
   6. Family and community resources.
   7. Immediate logistical problems and arrangements.

C. Offer encouragement regarding expected rehabilitation progress and the availability of assistance in returning to optimal level of functioning.

D. Assess client's interest in ongoing relationship.

Initial Family Contact

A. Initiate contact with family to introduce self and explain role.
B. Elicit any current concerns they wish to express.
C. Offer encouragement regarding expected rehabilitation progress.
D. Assist family in attaining full and realistic appreciation of anticipated physical and functional changes and their impact.
E. Elicit information pertinent to psychosocial issues which may impact on overall rehabilitation.
F. Assess family's interest in ongoing relationship

Post-Initial Treatment or Second Contact

Immediate Post-Op/Treatment Review

A. Contact physician to update pertinent information; i.e., pathology reports, surgical procedures performed, other treatment initiated, and general condition.
B. Visit client offering support even though client may be unable to communicate verbally. Assist him in expressing concerns, including:
   1. Perception of outcomes from surgery/other treatment.
   2. Response to institution and staff (if hospitalized).
   3. Perception of family reaction.
   4. Response to altered body image (real or imagined) and functional changes.
C. Reinforce positive coping strategies.
D. Provide for education and information in response to misperceptions or overreactions regarding normal course of events.

Pre-Discharge or Re-Integration into Primary Social Unit

Assessment/Treatment

A. Reinforce client's understanding of ongoing medical treatment plan (including physical and psychosocial rehabilitation).
B. Assess client's understanding of anticipated activity level.
C. Assist client in anticipation of resumption of previous or alternative roles, including family, social, sexual, and vocational aspects.
D. Determine that arrangements have been made for discharge and that needed resources have been identified.
E. Assist family in expressing concerns, including:
   1. Perception of treatment outcome.
   2. Perception of client's adjustment.
   3. Reaction to physical and functional changes.
   4. Perception of client's ability to resume previous or alternative roles, including family, social, sexual, and vocational aspects.
F. Reinforce positive coping strategies.
G. Provide for education and information in response to overreactions or unrealistic expectations family may have about client's functional capabilities.
H. Reinforce family's understanding of ongoing medical plan (including physical and psychological rehabilitation).

Post-Discharge or Pre-Employment

Post-Discharge Assessment/Treatment

A. Provide an opportunity for client to give comprehensive account of physical and social progress since discharge which may include:
   1. Degree of self-care.
   2. Extent of household responsibilities.
   3. Resumption of socializing with friends, community participation in family roles and activities.
B. Support areas of positive attempts towards goals. Encourage additional attempts and offer suggestions for alternative means to attain subsequent roles.

Post Discharge

C. Respond to current concerns, including:
   1. Perception of family relationships.
   2. Sexual role.
   3. Altered body and self-image.
   4. Physical disability.
   5. Obstacles to employment.
D. Reinforce realistic, positive feelings and correct misconceptions.
E. Reinforce positive coping strategies.
F. Support areas of positive family coping and adjustment attempts. Encourage supportive behavior and provide suggestions for alternative solution.

G. Respond to current concerns of family, such as:
1. Client's return to home milieu.
2. Altered family roles and patterns.
3. Physical disability and altered body appearance.
4. Sexual roles and communication.
5. Availability of resources, i.e., transportation and finances.

Adaptedby Fusco from Protocols developed by the Medical College of Virginia Cancer Rehabilitation Program under contract with the National Cancer Institute (NOI–CN–65287) (Fusco, 1978—slightly modified)

Employment Discrimination

Rehabilitation counseling emphasizes vocational goals, but closely related is the specific area of employment and reemployment rights. A number of disciplines are concerned with client advocacy but perhaps this concern is most often expressed by rehabilitation counselors, social workers, and legal aid personnel.

The Federal Rehabilitation Act provides protection for all handicapped persons, including those with a cancer diagnosis. The act pertains primarily to employers receiving federal funds. In some states, however, legislators and patient advocates have promoted anti-discrimination laws specifically for cancer patients. Many states have adopted supplemental state legislation to protect the rights of persons with disabilities. In New Jersey, for example, the State's Division of Civil Rights defends handicapped persons in court against job discrimination.

Most states have human rights laws which make separate legislation unnecessary. Cancer activists feel, however, that employment discrimination continues to be widespread against people with cancer histories, and that a separate law would highlight and clarify the need to eliminate such discrimination. Barbara Hoffman, spokesperson for the **National Coalition for Cancer Survivorship,** feels that using general laws that protect disabled persons perpetuates a negative stereotype of cancer survivors as chronically handicapped, when in fact many fully recover.

Recently many cancer survivors have been carrying their plea to the media. In 1985 Timothy Calonita, a 24-year-old New Yorker, was rejected as a police applicant by the Nassau County Civil Service because he had had Hodgkin's disease when he was 11 years old. Following years of appeals, and much local media publicity, Calonita was finally cleared for police work; civil service officials cited an "individual exception."

The New York Times has reported that both blue and white collar workers who are former cancer patients are routinely denied employment due to medical history, despite legislation in 37 states prohibiting such discrimination. There are also many reports of workers who were fired once management learned of a present or past cancer diagnosis. Thousands of workers are denied promotion, isolated from co-workers, and written-off in terms of new job opportunities since they are considered "not worth the investment" (*New York Times* 1 April 1984). In what is sometimes a well-meaning attempt to avoid straining energy levels, colleagues stop asking persons with a cancer history to take on difficult or challenging assignments.

Charges of discrimination are very hard to prove and very costly to litigate. Although laws are on the books, they are frequently ignored; consequently, the discrimination goes unchallenged.

In a *United Press International* release (19 May 1980) it was reported that a plumbing foreman attempted suicide when he was demoted after surgery for throat cancer. His subordinates mimicked his new way of speaking and the boss thought the foreman would not be able to regain their respect. Another cancer patient was fired because his boss feared he would be absent too much. When he applied for a new job he was asked to fill out an application with a pencil rather than a pen so that the pencil could be discarded. A woman who had undergone a mastectomy three years earlier was refused a library aide job on the recommendation of an examining physician.

A professor at the University of Southern California in social work, Frances Lomas Feldman, cited these and other examples of discrimination against persons with a cancer history. Ms. Feldman reports that a study of white collar workers revealed 54 percent of 127 persons interviewed experienced work related problems—including loss of job; refusal of promotion; and changes in salary, working conditions, hours, and insurance coverage—which were related to a cancer diagnosis. Among blue collar workers, the figure jumped to an astounding 84 percent.

Prominant people, such as former Indiana Senator Birch Bayh, are beginning to speak out against cancer discrimination in the work place. In a recent *New York Times* article written by Senator Bayh, he publicized some of the work done by Dr. Feldman and others. Bayh cites the positive experiences of employers like the Metropolitan Life Insurance Company and American Telephone and Telegraph Company. Both found that work performance, absenteeism, and turnover were comparable for people with and without cancer histories.

In a study of the social, economic, and psychological needs of California cancer patients, the illness was found to have profound effects on the person's employment future. Fewer than 35 percent of the patients in the study were still working for the employer they had before they were diagnosed, and there was a strong positive correlation between level of income and those who were working for the same employer. Some patients reported that the net effect of their illness was to lock them into their former jobs. If they were to change jobs, they feared losing hospital and other medical insurance, pension rights, and other benefits.

Employees in highly skilled positions reported the fewest problems in returning to former jobs. Perhaps employers recognized they were protecting an investment in welcoming workers back. The study did not disclose whether those who did not return to work were fired or forced into early retirement (American Cancer Society, California Div., 1979).

In a country like the United States, people are judged by the work they do. The work ethic and high value on self-reliance remain high in American priorities.

Psychotherapy

Various forms of counseling have been covered in this book. Among the deepest, most intense forms of counseling is psychotherapy. Closely related to, and in some cases indistinguishable from, psychological counseling, psychotherapy traditionally is a longer process. Counseling is generally regarded as more cognitive than psychotherapy. The techniques used are somewhat different, and those may differ from therapist to therapist. Both counseling and psychotherapy strive to bring about change in the client/patient, and both are aimed at fostering development. A review of the earlier section of *Crucial Components of Counseling Practice* will provide the reader with some other commonly made distinctions between counseling and psychotherapy as well as some of the philosophic and theoretical differences among the various schools of thought.

Considering the vast amount that has been written about psychotherapy and about persons with cancer, not much has been written about psychotherapeutic counseling for persons with cancer. Perhaps the most comprehensive review of the subject to date was done by Jane Goldberg (1981) in her book *Psychotherapeutic Treatment of Cancer Patients.*

Goldberg points out at the outset that psychological intervention is still an experimental and adjunctive form of treatment for persons with cancer. When medical science finds the answer or answers to this disease, some forms of counseling and therapy may be no longer needed. She believes that until then, full exploration of the possible value of psychotherapy should be continued.

Goldberg invited a number of workers in the field of psychotherapy to contribute to a very readable book she edited and to which she herself contributed several sections explaining some of her personal experiences and views. In one of her sections entitled "Theoretical Considerations" she points out that cancer "has been seen alternatively as a virus, a lowering of immunological defenses, a biochemical imbalance caused by nutritional deficiencies, a breakdown of cellular communication, a characterological defense against aggression, a resistance to a positive transference to a psychoanalyst, a somatization of pre-oedipal impulses, a freezing of energy and more" (Goldberg, 1981, p. 1.)

In discussing the possibility of a psychosomatic component in the development of cancer, Goldberg (1981) states that researchers have validated a personality profile of the cancer patient, which includes three major traits: repression of feeling, inhibition of aggression, and an extremely pleasant personality.

In the same work, Herbert Bilick and William Nuland describe a psychological model in treating cancer patients. In working with groups of cancer patients they find it useful for patients to develop meaningful and realistic goals to enhance the quality of life. They also stress the importance of family support systems. In special group meetings, family members are assisted in identifying long-standing, unresolved conflicts (Goldberg, 1981, pp. 63–64).

Bilick and Nuland also discuss the difficult problems of dealing with recurrence and death:

In the event of a recurrence, patients are encouraged to give themselves enough time (at least two weeks) to grapple with the meaning of the recurrence and to make a conscious choice of whether they want to continue to fight or whether they feel it is time to die. A patient may feel that his physical deterioration and emotional anguish are too great an obstacle to overcome and that it would be better to say his last goodbyes to his family and friends. For patients who decide to give up in this way, their death, although painful for the family, leaves fewer psychological scars and unresolved issues because all concerned are given the opportunity to express their deepest feelings to one another during the final separation. It is important to remember that the majority of patients continue to fight at these crossroads but that they now fight as a result of choice rather then out of guilt, family obligation, or unexpressed fears (Goldberg, 1981, pp. 64–65).

Carl and Stephanie Simonton's work in the areas of self-hypnosis, imagery, and visualization will be discussed later in this work when self-help techniques are covered. But it might be briefly mentioned here that the Simontons' methods often are professionally guided, and accompanied by, individual and group psychotherapy. The Simontons reported some statistics concerning Stage IV terminal patients which suggest the possibility that psychological treatment intervention can contribute to remission, can slow tumor growth, and can raise activity levels among some patients.

Dr. Larry Le Shan is a well-known therapist who has done considerable work with cancer patients using individual psychotherapy. He believes that patients can improve both physically and in terms of quality of life if they receive psychotherapy. Goldberg clearly agrees, and has advanced the theory that psychological factors not only can contribute to the healing or worsening of a malignant condition, but are also important contributors to the initial development of the cancer. A "loss-depression" concept is discussed which suggests that persons who have lost an important object—an important relationship, for example, or a material possession—can place a person at higher risk for developing a malignancy. The "cancer personality" theory mentioned earlier is also discussed by Goldberg in the context of treating cancer as a psychosomatic disease. In general, a cancer-prone person is described as an individual who represses emotions, especially anger (Goldberg, 1981, p. 71).

Richard Renneker contributed what may be one of the most valuable chapters to Goldberg's book, for the patient as well as the practitioner. Renneker examines many issues related to psychotherapy and cancer. He seems to be feeling his way, along with us the readers, in a search for some answers. Although admitting to having a strong positive opinion about the power of psychological and emotional states as potential agents in disease (and in resistance to disease), he confides that as he has worked with individual patients he has often changed his methods and his thinking. Renneker believes that many threatening thoughts associated with cancer—such as death, helplessness, hopelessness, and loss of control—are very difficult for therapists to deal with. He believes also that the literature is convincing in describing personality features and life situations of cancer patients, such as:

- cold and remote parents
- denial and repression of negative emotions, particularly anger
- lack of self-assertiveness and self-fullness
- helplessness and hopelessness
- despair and depression
- inability to cope successfully with a severe emotional loss (Goldberg, 1981, p. 144).

Renneker focuses on the pleasantness of cancer patients, labeling it a "pathological niceness syndrome." He relates this to the alleged cancer personality feature of denying and repressing negative feelings, particularly anger. Persons who grow up without rebelling against parents develop pathological niceness, contends Renneker. He believes that therapists need to teach cancer patients the ineffectiveness and harmfulness of being indiscriminately nice and for patients to learn patterns of self assertiveness. Patients need to be taught active ways of being helpful in their own behalf so they can prevent hopelessness from developing. A therapist might, for example, help a patient prepare a list of questions to ask his surgeon.

The concept of a "cancer personality" is controversial and does not receive universal support among counselors. Many persons with cancer are offended, and even outraged, at many of the assertions made by writers like Goldberg and Renneker. A fuller discussion of this issue appears in a later section of this book entitled, *Seeking Personality Change.*

Renneker admits that not all cancer patients he has encountered fit into the model described. He believes that for those who are "pathologically nice" and fall into the helplessness-hopelessness pattern, therapeutic intervention is critical. If a patient is definitely terminal, Renneker emphasizes developing coping skills more and fighting skills less. Through his association with a special psychoanalytic project at a California hospital he identified a number of things that he became convinced are anti-therapeutic. Some of them have particular relevance for therapists working with cancer patients.

1. The sick patient and the healthy analyst attitude.
2. Therapist failure to provide a healthy, human model for the patient and refusal to provide any personal information about the therapist's beliefs, standards, and life experiences.

3. Interpreting patient's remarks as transference rather then recognizing them as analyst's countertransference behavior.
4. Therapist's need to have the patient agree with him.
5. Therapist's lack of respect for patients; as evidenced by therapists speaking like an all-knowing parent speaking to a beligerent child.
6. Therapist's failure to provide appreciation feedback to patient; therapist enjoys having the patient make positive statements about him but rarely responds in kind.
7. Therapist's distortions; as seen particularly in faulty memory of what the patient actually said. (Goldberg, 1981, pp 158–9).

Michael Kerr, also a contributor to Jane Goldberg's book, emphasized the importance of the family unit in treating a person with cancer. Surprisingly, he cautions the therapist **against** focusing on feeling. His view is that there is enough feeling permeating the cancer environment without the therapist pushing "to get the feelings out." He would rather have the therapist listen calmly to what people are thinking. This low-key attitude is not intended to mask feelings or to encourage denial, but rather to create a relaxed, light atmosphere in which emotion is controlled and family members can deal with the issues at hand. Kerr asserts that most failures in cancer therapy are the result of the therapist not recognizing and adequately diffusing the emotional intensity of the sessions (Goldberg, 1981, pp 309–310).

Chapter 6

PATIENTS HELPING THEMSELVES—
AN EXAMINATION OF
SELF-HEALING THEORY AND METHODS

Patients, especially persons with serious illnesses, often feel passive and helpless. They are put in the position of waiting to receive assistance from others. Many succumb to a fatalistic attitude and a passive "help me, please" view of both their future and life in general. Fortunately this is sometimes just a phase, a reaction to the shock of illness, and is not permanent. Many patients rouse themselves out of this helpless, passive mode and begin to try to fight the illness, or at least have some impact on its course.

A widely used resource for self-motivation and self-instruction is the written word. Although many persons with cancer do not seek the services of a counselor, they will read published materials about the illness. As discussed in an earlier section of this work, many pamphlets and booklets are published by both government and private sources, especially the American Cancer Society and the National Institutes of Health. Books and, with increasing frequency, audio tapes are used by thousands of cancer patients to guide them through the dizzying variety of orthodox and unorthodox treatment options available today.

MEDITATION, RELAXATION AND MENTAL IMAGERY

Books focusing on "self-help" and "self-healing" have become increasingly popular. These books generally promote the idea that the patient can influence the course of his or her illness through the power of the mind. Mental processes are described which are thought by many to promote relaxation and a feeling of well-being.

Carl Simonton has been in the forefront of this movement for nearly a decade. His book, *Getting Well Again* (1978), written with Stephanie Mathews Simonton and James Creighton, is perhaps the most well-known reference source for the mind-body approach to cancer treatment. It has given comfort and hope to untold numbers of cancer patients.

The Simontons established a treatment facility in the Southwest where many cancer patients have gone to learn and practice the techniques of meditation, relaxation, and mental imagery. Audio tapes may be purchased with either Carl or Stephanie leading the patient in a series of relaxation, and mental imagery exercises. Simple breathing exercises and focused meditation usually begin the process; learning to relax muscle groups in the body is often the next step. The exercises eventually guide the patient to mentally picture weak, confused cancer cells being attacked and overtaken by vigorous, aggressive treatment forms, represented by images such as sharks, Pac-Man type aggressors, or swords symbolizing the body's white blood cells. The body's determined immune system is seen as attacking and engulfing the disorganized cancer cells. The Simontons suggest a routine of practicing imagery of this type three times a day, and they enthusiastically report encouraging results. Published studies indicate tumor regression for some patients, disease stabilization for others and even disease remission for a substantial portion (22 percent of the survivors).

The surviving patients are said to have exceeded the national average by two times for living after cancer diagnosis (Appelbaum in Goldberg, 1981). Reportedly all these patients had been pronounced incurable. As Appelbaum points out (in Goldberg, 1981) the statistics must be considered in the light of special factors, primarily the personality characteristics of patients who seek out unconventional treatments. They are more likely to be fighters, persons who are more likely to emerge as "survivors." It is safe to say that such persons are, at the very least, highly motivated. Despite being in poor health, many of them needed to travel some distance, often at considerable cost, to participate in a new and unproven treatment.

Appelbaum talks also of a possible "placebo effect"; i.e., the suggestibility of the whole technique. People are, in a sense, undergoing hypnotherapy in a warm, caring, optimistic environment.

SEEKING PERSONALITY CHANGE

In the Goldberg edition, *Psychotherapeutic Treatment of Cancer Patients,* Appelbaum describes his personal and professional affiliation with the Simontons. He openly admits that he was a most biased researcher,

wanting very much to believe in the effectiveness of psychological treatment in curing cancer. Although he lacked objectivity and employed
some sloppy research methodology, he became convinced that personality
characteristics do play a role in either the etiology or the course of cancer.
He describes, in anecdotal fashion, his extended psychotherapeutic work
with several patients and calls for more controlled experimentation, with
long-term psychotherapy used as a treatment for the disease. He does
not report encouraging results in terms of survival, or even in the
amelioration of symptoms.

What is disturbing to many scientists and cancer patients is the
implication in this type of work that the patient is responsible for
developing his or her disease and that he or she will be doubly guilty if a
self-cure fails. As Goldberg points out in the introductory section of her
book, illness can be viewed as the end product of "a characterological
deficiency" (1981 p xxv). The early fundamentalists advanced the notion
that sickness is a punishment for evil behavior. Variations of that theme
still emerge today, although in a more subtle and sophisticated form.
The whole notion of a "cancer personality" has not substantial support
in any of the literature; yet the myth continues to be embellished. The
idea of shy, withdrawn people predominating among cancer patients
appears in the literature as a hypothesis based on some clinical observations of a few people (those who don't fit the mold are mentally discarded),
and is picked up by other writers and researchers, who spread the myth
further. What is needed, perhaps, is some independent thinking by
today's counselors and psychotherapists. They must be willing to look at
the totality of the population, without prejudice and without relying on
others' hypotheses or their bold and premature conclusions. The primary
reason that unbiased and independent thinking is needed is simply that
practitioners and writers do a great disservice to people who are trying
to restore normalcy to their lives by spreading myths and unsupported
theories. The "cancer personality" type of myth can promote feelings of
guilt and helplessness, and it can become a self-fulfilling prophesy.
Premature conclusions should clearly be withheld until stronger evidence is available to either support or debunk the theory.

This writer's beliefs are clearly on the side of a conservative and
cautious approach to any conclusions about personality characteristics
in either the development or cure of cancer. In the interests of a comprehensive and fair presentation, however, the views of people who feel
differently have been included. This does not mean that such methods

as meditation and visualization are not useful for cancer patients. On the contrary, they have reportedly helped many persons to feel better and to improve their quality of life. As useful self-help techniques, these methods are enthusiastically endorsed. The cautionary note is reserved for the leap to unsubstantiated conclusions about a common set of personality characteristics among cancer patients, about the psychoanalytic interpretations of how these characteristics developed, and about the assertions concerning substantially affecting the course or outcome of the disease process through therapeutic intervention.

HYPNOTHERAPY

A logical extension of the discussion of meditation, relaxation, and visualization is hypnotherapy. Although hypnotherapy is often thought of as therapy administered by a trained hypnotist, it can be—with instruction and practice—a self-healing technique. As with meditation and relaxation and mental imagery, a personal, professional guide, or at least a good instructional book, is needed in the early stages.

Hypnotic induction techniques, such as arm levitation, eye fixation, and deep muscle relaxation, are all geared toward changing the consciousness state. Focusing attention should assist movement into a more relaxed state, facilitating visualization and suggestibility. The patient can be taught to put himself into a trance state, and to make life-enhancing suggestions to himself. Autohypnosis is often helpful in coping with fear and pain as well (Goldberg, 1981).

The reader may recognize that much of the material discussed in this section and in the preceding sections can be traced to yoga and to Eastern philosophy and beliefs.

BIOFEEDBACK

For some time now medical and social science personnel have worked toward improving health by providing feedback of physical indicators to patients. Typically, a tense, so-called Type A personality will be taught methods of relaxation, and then be hooked up to machines to monitor breathing rate, body temperature, blood pressure, etc. As the patient strives to relax, he observes the figures of his vital signs on machines before him. In many cases this feedback information allows the patient to achieve healthier readings.

The biofeedback trainer might, for example, have a patient think about warming his hands as a method of ceasing a migraine headache. As the patient succeeds in "thinking his hands (or even a single finger) warmer," temperature readings will record the degree of his success. That people can learn to do this is indisputable. Just how the migraine ceases is not clear, but it has been suggested that the headache disappears because blood is diverted from the brain to the extremities.

Critics may say that patient scores are artificially inflated at the start since many people will react with high stress to having all sorts of monitors attached to them. When the patient becomes familiar with the setting and begins to calm down, medical improvement is claimed. Also the possible influence of temporary distraction needs to be mentioned as leading to scores that may be spuriously good. The major question is whether or not the experience is transferable to other times of the day, out of the artificial laboratory-like atmosphere of the training session.

Nonetheless, advocates of this method of self-healing proclaim its value not only for cancer, but also for heart disease, hypertension, and many other stress-related disorders. Because many patients report positive results it should be regarded as a legitimate treatment. Biofeedback normally requires a teacher, often a nurse-therapist or a specially trained social worker, to work with the patient. Eventually the patient can be taught to continue without assistance.

EXERCISE

Exercise has been suggested as a prevention and a cure for many physical ailments, including cancer. A certain breed of cancer patient feels that physical activity is an effective way to deal with the various negative feelings that cancer brings on.

There are different types of exercise regimens, of course. The type of exercise discussed here is not physical therapy a post-mastectomy patient is advised to follow to regain muscular control and strength. Believers in the fitness movement include cancer patients like Ruth Heidrich, who finished second in her age division in a grueling triathlon (*Newsday*, 20 Nov. 1986). Exercise has become her means of coping. Even after a second cancer surgery, the 51-year-old grandmother continued to cycle 350 miles, run 75 miles, and swim 7 miles weekly.

Some researchers, such as researchers at Ohio State University's Comprehensive Cancer Center, are investigating the effect of exercise on cancer patients. In 1981 the Department of Behavioral Medicine and Psychiatry in Charlottesville, Virginia, reported on the use of exercise in the prevention and treatment of cancer. In personal correspondence with the writer, Robert S. Brown, Ph.D., M.D., Director of that study, explained the rationale for such explorations.

> Some years ago I discovered a feeling of well-being associated with physical fitness. This discovery led me to take a new look at my practice of psychiatry whereupon I discovered I had rarely, if ever treated a physically fit psychiatric patient. Soon thereafter, I started encouraging my psychiatric patients to exercise, particularly walking, to see if it would help them with their depression and anxiety. The results have been overwhelmingly in favor of exercise. About one year ago, it occurred to me that people who are physically fit may have a greater resistance to environmental carcinogins. With the help of the University of Virginia Oncology Clinic, I discussed the possibility of encouraging patients with cancer to begin a walking program to see if this would help reduce some of their stress. The results to date have been favorable. (Brown, 1981)

Some observers have objected to putting weak, frightened cancer patients through painful and taxing exercise regimens. It would indeed be insensitive and cruel to promote difficult and excessive levels of exercise among seriously ill people without any real indication that such a regimen would be beneficial. In fact, this writer first corresponded with Dr. Brown to object to his study. However, the mild and undemanding exercise that Dr. Brown described in his reply can surely do no harm, and might even be of benefit to some people. Again, persons with cancer as well as workers in the field need to consider whether there is any potential value in incorporating exercise as part of their overall cancer treatment (or coping) program.

DIETARY APPROACHES

Much was said in an early section of this book on the possible role that nutrition plays in causing, preventing, and treating cancer. Diet needs to be mentioned again, however, to stress the great deal of recent attention that has been given to nutrition as a self-healing method for cancer patients.

Many people have reduced their intake of processed sugars, fats, red meats, and smoked fish products, and instead are eating vegetables, fruits, and low fat dairy products. Most nutritionists recommend whole grain products, monounsaturated fats and oils, poultry, and baked fish. Foods rich in Vitamin C are viewed by some as life-extending, even for patients with advanced cancer. Citrus fruits and yogurt have long been recommended as cancer-inhibiting foods.

Most health care workers do not endorse extremely limited diets, such as macrobiotics.

There is little evidence on therapeutic benefits of any diet in the treatment of cancer. Max Gerson, a German physician, offered a dietary regimen in the 1920s that limited all foods except fresh fruits, vegetables, and oatmeal. It still has some adherents today. Somewhat changed, the Gerson regimen now includes coffee enemas, frequent intake of fruit juices, castor and linseed oil supplements, vitamin B-12 injections, and other enzymes and minerals (*New York Times*, 7 December 1988).

Diet therapies are said to restore metabolic balance or detoxify the patient in some way. The greatest danger of such programs are that patients may fail to utilize conventional treatments available, having developed total faith in the dietary treatment. Cancer is best treated in its very earliest stages; delaying conventional treatment to try alternate forms of therapy can doom the patient to certain death.

Megadoses of nutrients can be very hazardous. Too much vitamin A or selenium is toxic. Large amounts of vitamin C can promote leukemia cell growth, according to Dr. Victor Herbert of the Mt. Sinai School of Medicine (*New York Times*, 7 December 1988).

LEARNING TO BE AN EXCEPTIONAL PATIENT

Many people believe that there is a direct connection between a robust will to live and the chemical balances in the brain. Norman Cousins is convinced of the negative effects of negative emotions on body chemistry. His famous book, *Anatomy of an Illness*, encourages love, hope, faith, laughter, confidence, and the will to live.

Dr. Bernie Siegel refers to the "exceptional" patient in his book *Love, Medicine and Miracles* (1986). By this he does not mean exceptionally good; in fact he encourages patients to be inquiring, complaining, demanding, and feisty, and even suggests that uncooperative or difficult patients are the ones most likely to get well. Siegel's writing stresses the role of physician as teacher. He reiterates the Simontons' positive outlook: "In the face of uncertainty, there is nothing wrong with hope."

Siegel describes some characteristics that he has observed among surviving patients. Independence and assertiveness are high on his list, and he believes that expressing loving feelings contributes to the healing process. His book takes the position that a "survivor" personality can be learned.

One might quibble with many of Siegel's unsupported conclusions and his effusive style is sometimes a bit extreme, but his book presents many ideas worth serious consideration. He has a warm and winning manner in his lectures and although he relies on much anecdotal material and emotional stories of a few unusual individuals who made miraculous recoveries from serious illness, the overall effect is inspiring. He could disarm and win over the crankiest and most skeptical audience.

DELIMITATIONS AND CAVEATS ABOUT SELF-HEALING

When people read about all the non-medical treatment options that are promoted for the cure and amelioration of cancer, they sometimes feel guilty about not making full use of all the alternatives available, or, worse, making use of them and still failing. It must be emphasized that the approaches discussed in this section are attempts to heal or improve life quality; they do not guarantee a cure. These approaches may not all work for all people.

The various psychological treatments have been of particular controversy. A study in Boston, reported in *The New England Journal of Medicine*, disputes the notion that a positive mental attitude helps to fight disease. As has been discussed at length in this book, many mental health workers maintain that people who are hopeless and passive when confronted by serious illness are more likely to die, while fighters tend to survive. When tested objectively, however, no support for this assertion was found (*New York Times*, 13 June 1985). The study was done with people having advanced cancer, and it was concluded that their personalities, social lives, and way of life were unrelated to their survival. Reactions to the study have led some practitioners to conclude that psychological factors **may** play some role, but it is not a simple or certain one. Perhaps it is a limited role, one which is greatly influenced by many other factors (*The Record*, 13 June 1987). Other researchers have insisted that for certain types of tumors behavior may be a biological modifier. The danger in assuming a cause and effect relationship between psychological factors and cancer is that some patients may shun conventional treatment methods and focus instead on psychotherapy or relaxation or mental imagery. Dr. Marcia Angell, of *The New England Journal of Medicine*, wrote in an accompanying editorial: "It is time to acknowledge that our belief in disease as a direct reflection of mental state is largely folklore." People need not and should not feel that they are in any way to blame for their illness, nor that they lack optimal self-discipline or the will to live.

Similarly, many ill people develop unnecessary guilt about long-established eating patterns, especially members of ethnic cultures that have traditionally had high fat or meat consumption in their diet, when they read that their eating traditions are not in conformity with recent pronouncements about proper diet.

Our knowledge about many of the self-healing approaches discussed in this section are still in a primitive stage. Merely having a good attitude is not enough to change the course of a devastating disease. We need to remind ourselves, and those we work with, that cancer is not a punishment for a "loser mentality," for wrong thinking, or for a weak will to live. It is pointless and insensitive to imply that people could cure themselves if they would only try harder. We may learn, however, that patients who actively participate in their treatment programs and who maintain a degree of control over what is happening to them may indeed fare better, even if it is just a little better for just a limited period of time. Faith, hope, and an assertive positive attitude cannot hurt, and, if little else, will surely make the illness easier to bear.

SUMMARY

This book has reviewed the field of counseling, including the critical components of counseling practice. No single counseling orientation or style is correct for all practitioners but, when a style is chosen, the practitioner must develop a philosophy and a fidelity to his or her beliefs. Various helpful counseling techniques can be learned, and, with practice, perfected.

A primer to understanding cancer was presented with the hope that, although considerable information was provided, it was explained in a manner understandable to laymen. Various causal factors, as well as the state of the art in treatment methods, were discussed at length.

In an attempt to put these two bodies of knowledge together, the culminating section was devoted to counseling persons with cancer. The author drew widely on his own experience in this area, and attempted to describe in detail the emotional state of the person with cancer. He described the common feelings, emotional stages, and family reactions, as he has observed them over the past several years.

A central theme of this work is that there are many different types of counseling, performed by persons with varying backgrounds. The specialties discussed included counseling performed by clergy, peer counseling offered by persons who have themselves had the disease, rehabilitation counseling, and psychotherapy.

Finally, various self-healing methods were described and examined, including meditation, mental imagery, deep muscle relaxation, hypnotherapy, biofeedback, nutritional treatments, and exercise.

Although the author made no attempt to hide his own counseling philosophy, beliefs, and biases, an attempt was made to fairly present all sides of controversial issues and practices.

Exciting new developments, and some minor breakthroughs, occurred in the field of cancer research in the time it took to prepare this manuscript. A study reported in *The New York Times* only a week before the writer began the final draft tied a genetic defect to a form of cancer. This discovery is expected to lead to better understanding of a certain type of lung cancer, which accounts for at least 20 percent of all lung cancers. Similarly, new approaches in the treatment of bladder cancer have been reported in the very recent past. Cancer of the colon has also been in the spotlight recently. Scientists in England have found strong evidence of a genetic defect linked to colon cancer. This development may make it possible to detect a predisposition to cancer of the colon. Within a year of this writing the Dana-Farber Cancer Institute reported that it has had highly promising results using bone marrow transplants for non-Hodgkin's B-cells lymphoma, the most common form of tumor in young adults. In an experimental study, 65 percent of those patients treated survived this very virulent form of malignancy.

A gene associated with the development of cancer in laboratory experiments has recently been shown to be activated in lung cancer tissue. Scientists believe this gene may be a factor in developing the malignancy. The Netherlands Cancer Institute reported this suspected genetic link to lung cancer in a recent issue of *The New England Journal of Medicine.* Also during the period of this writing, a new and improved method for assessing the effectiveness of treatment for prostate cancer was developed at Stanford University.

At the Cold Spring Harbor Laboratory in Laurel Hollow, New York, biologist Ed Harlow and his colleagues have discovered that so called oncogenes may not cause tumors directly. Rather, they may shut off a bodily system that guards against cancer by preventing cells from growing too fast. If the protective gene's effect is blocked, uncontrolled growth, and hence cancer, begins. This subtle molecular mechanism provides important insight into how normal cells are converted into cancer cells.

Speaking in New Orleans at the 79th annual meeting of the American Association for Cancer Research, Dr. Isaiah J. Fidler of the M.D. Anderson Hospital and Tumor Institute in Houston, Texas, revealed his significant finding that migrating cancer cells are programmed to grow only in certain tissues. Only one cell in 100,000 released by a tumor is capable of beginning a cancer colony in a new site. Metastasis is beginning to be understood as a highly regulated process.

Although we sometimes feel that this scourge of humankind will be with us forever, and that forward movement occurs with glacially slow progress, it is encouraging to note these advances recorded by the media just during the relatively short time it took to complete this book.

We know that an attitude of hopefulness and positive expectation can be helpful during times of adversity. Cancer patients, their families and friends, and those who counsel them, need to remind themselves and each other of the progress that has been made and will be made. While we wait for the ultimate breakthrough in solving the mysteries of cancer let us help each other to do what we can to restore health, and to develop whatever coping skills work for us and for those who trust in our care.

REFERENCES

American Cancer Society. *Sixth National Cancer Conference Proceedings.* Philadelphia and Toronto: Lippincott, 1970.

American Cancer Society. *Answering Your Questions About Cancer.* New York: American Cancer Society, 1971, Reprinted 1974.

American Cancer Society. *The Hopeful Side of Cancer.* New York: ACS, 1976.

American Cancer Society, California Division. *Report on the Social, Economic and Psychological Needs of Cancer Patients in California.* San Francisco: ACS, 1979.

American Cancer Society. *Cancer Facts and Figures.* New York American Cancer Society, 1987.

Berg, John W. "Nutrition and Cancer," in *Understanding Cancer.* ed. Renneker, Mark and Lieb, Steven. Palo Alto, California: Bull Publishing, 1979.

Biggs, Marcia, "Opening the dating game to people with handicaps," *The Detroit News,* reprinted in *Newsday* (New York) 2 April 1985, Part II, p. 7.

Bateson, Gregory. *Mind and Nature: A Necessary Unity.* New York: Bantam, 1980.

Blocher, Donald. *Developmental Counseling.* New York: Ronald Press, 1966.

Bolton, Brian, and Jacques, Marcelline. *Rehabilitation Counseling: Theory and Practice.* Baltimore: University Park Press, 1978.

Bordin, Edward S. *Psychological Counseling.* New York: Appleton-Century-Crofts, 1955.

Bowen, Murray. *Family Therapy in Clinical Practice.* New York: Jason Arenson, 1978.

Boyd, William. *The Spontaneous Regression of Cancer.* New York: Charles C Thomas, 1966.

Brayfield, A. H. *Readings in Modern Methods of Counseling.* New York: Appleton-Century-Crofts, 1950.

Brickner, Abraham. "Action for Reducing Barriers to Employment and Community Participation" *The Role of Vocational Rehabilitation in the 1980's.* Perlman, L. (ed.) Washington, D.C.: N.R.A., 1978, pp. 1–13.

Brown, Robert S. Personal letter, 16, March 1981.

Buchheimer, Arnold and Balogh, Sara Carter. *The Counseling Relationship.* Chicago: Science Research Associates, 1961.

Bush, Haydn. "Cancer, the New Synthesis—Cure," *Science 84,* September 1984, pp. 34–35.

Ca—A Cancer Journal for Clinicians. "Unproven Methods of Cancer Management—Macrobiotic Diets," Vol. 34, No. 1, January/February 1984, pp. 60–63.

Callis; Polmantier; Roeber. *A Casebook of Counseling.* New York: Appleton-Century-Crofts, 1955.

Cameron, Ewan and Pauling, Linus. *Cancer and Vitamin C.* Menlo Park, California: Linus Pauling Institute of Science and Medicine, 1979.

Cantor, Robert. *And a Time to Live.* New York: Harper Colophon Books, 1980.

Clark, Matt; Morris, Holly; King, Patricia; Abramson, Pamela; Gosnell, Marian; Hager, Mary; Burgower, Barbara; Huck, Janet; "Living With Cancer," *Newsweek,* 8 April 1985.

Clark, Matt; Shapiro, Dan and Friendly, David T. "Cancer—A Progress Report," *Newsweek,* 3 November 1979.

Clark, Matt; Shapiro, Dan and Friendly, David T. "Cancer—A Progress Report," *Newsweek,* 2 November 1981.

Coggle, J.E. *Biological Effects of Radiation.* New York: Wykeham, 1971.

Cohn, Victor. "Progress in Cancer War Noted," *The Washington Post,* 29 November 1983.

Conti, John V. "Vocational Rehabilitation," *Living With Cancer,* Vol. 4, No. 5, November 1981, p. 1.

Conti, John V. "Independent Living," *Living With Cancer,* Vol. 5, No. 1, February 1982, p. 1.

Corey, G. *Theory and Practice of Counseling and Psychotherapy.* (3rd Edition). Monteray, California: Brooks-Cole, 1986.

Cousins, Norman. *Anatomy of an Illness.* New York: W.W. Norton, 1979.

Cox, B. G. "The fine art of educating the patient," *Medical Opinion.* 4:31–35, 1975.

Cox, B. G., Carr, D. T., and Lee, R. E. *Living with Lung Cancer: A Reference Book for People with Lung Cancer and Their Families.* Rochester, Minn.: Mayo Foundation, 1977.

Crawford, Donald H. Jr. "A Needs Assessment Inventory for Rehabilitation Agency Personnel," Unpublished taxonomy of rehabilitation training needs undertaken at the Continuing Education Program for Rehabilitation, State University of New York at Buffalo, 1987.

Edwards, Deanna. "Music, Laughter, and Tears," a talk delivered at *the Ninth Annual Patient Education Conference: Living with Cancer—New Horizons IX,* Sponsored by the American Cancer Society, Long Island Chapter, at the Adelphi Huntington Center, Huntington Station, New York, 10 June 1987.

Estes, Jane. *Pasadena Star News.* Pasadena, California, 1980, reprinted in brochure *We Can Do!—A Unique Cancer Support Group,* 1981.

Feinberg, Arthur M. "Observations—On Being Healthily Skeptical," *Newsday* (New York), 4 April 1985.

Fiedler, Fred E. "The Concept of an Ideal Therapeutic Relationship," *Journal of Consulting Psychology,* XIV, August 1950, pp. 239–45.

Fiedler, Fred E. "A Comparison of Therapeutic Relationships in Psychoanalytic, Non-Directive and Adlerian Therapy," *Journal of Consulting Psychology,* XIV, December 1950, pp. 436–45.

Franco, Patricia C. (ed.) *The Challenge of Cancer Rehabilitation: A Handbook for Vocational Rehabilitation Counselors.* Richmond, Virginia: Virginia Commonwealth University, 1978.

Goldberg, Jane G. (ed.) *Psychotherapeutic Treatment of Cancer Patients.* New York: The Free Press, 1981.

Healey, John E., Jr., and Zilis, Jack. "Cancers" in *Handbook of Severe Disability,* Stolov, W.C. and Clowers, M.R. (eds.) Washington, D.C.: U.S. Govt. Printing Office, 1981, pp. 363–375.

Heidenstam, David. "Cancer," in *Man's Body: An Owner's Manual.* New York: Paddington Press Ltd., 1976.

Jaffe, Dennis. *Healing from Within.* New York: Alfred A. Knopf, 1980.

Kelly, Orville. *Until Tomorrow Comes.* New York: Everest House, 1979.

Krant, Melvin J. "Action for Improving Socialization and Family Support, and Reducing Stigma and Negative Attitudes," in *The Role of Vocational Rehabilitation in the 1980's: Serving Those With Invisible Handicaps.* Perlman, L. (ed.) Washington, D.C.: N.R.A., 1978, pp. 15–30.

LeShan, Lawrence. *You Can Fight For Your Life.* New York: Harcourt, Brace, Javanovich, 1977.

Matkin, R. E. "The roles and functions of rehabilitation specialists in the private sector." *Journal of Applied Rehabilitation Counseling,* 14(1), 1983, pp. 14–27.

McAleer, C. A. "Cancer: a rehabilitation challenge," *Journal of Applied Rehabilitation Counseling,* Vol. 6, 1975, pp. 83–87.

McGowan, John F., (ed.), *An Introduction to the Vocational Rehabilitation Process.* U.S. Dept. of H.E.W., GTP Bulletin No. 3, Rehabilitation Service Series No. 555, Washington, D.C.: U.S. Govt. Printing Office, 1980.

McKay, Diane. "Viruses and Cancer," in *Understanding Cancer* ed. Renneker, Mark and Lieb, Steven. Palo Alto, California: Bull, 1979.

McLaughlin, W. J. "Cancer rehabilitation: people investing in people," *Journal of Rehabilitation,* 50(4), 57–59, 1984.

Moses, H., Borell, K., Siler, A. "Issues in developing peer counseling programs," *Conference Proceedings: Region VII Conference on Independent Living.* Lawrence, Kansas: Research and Training Center on Independent Living, 1982.

Moss, Rabbi Steven. "A Workshop on the Spiritual Needs of Cancer Patients," a talk delivered at *The Ninth Annual Patient Education Conference: Living with Cancer— New Horizons IX,* Sponsored by the American Cancer Society, Long Island Chapter, at the Adelphi Huntington Center, Huntington Station, New York, 10 June 1987.

Muthard, J. E. & Salamone, P. R. "The role and functions of the rehabilitation counselor." *Rehabilitation Counseling Bulletin,* 13, 1969, pp. 81–168.

New York Times, Lazarus, Barbara. "A Victim of Cancer; Then, of Employers," 1 April 1984.

New York Times, "Doubled Cancer Rate is Forecast," 21 April 1985.

New York Times, "Striking Change in Cancer Study," 9 December 1986.

New York Times, Schmeck, Harold M. "Cancer of Colon is Believed Linked to Defect in Gene," 13 August 1987, p. A1.

New York Times Schmeck, Harold M. "Study Ties Genetic Defect to Form of Lung Cancer," 1 October 1987, p. A17.

New York Times, "Treatment of Prostate Cancer," 8 October 1987, p. A28.

New York Times, "Scientists Link an Activated Gene to Lung Cancer," 8 October 1987, p. A28.

New York Times, Brody, Jane E. "Personal Health—Illusions and realities for patients who would fight cancer with dietary strategies," 7 December 1988.

New York University/Human Resources Center, Employment Research and Training Center RT-34. "Transition Resource Handbook for Parents and Professionals-Handbook I, Education and Vocation Issues" Family Research and Training Project. *The Least Restrictive Environment: Knowing One When You See It.* Reprinted from National Information Center for Handicapped Children and Youth, No. 5, 1985, p. 12.

Newsday, (New York), Zinman, David. "Evolving theories mark the search for cancer's cure," 6 April 1981, Part II, p. 9.

Newsday, (New York), Zinman, David. "Researchers Probe Heat as an Alternate Cancer Therapy," 21 September 1981, Part II, p. 8.

Newsday, (New York), Colen, B. D. "The lab, not the clinic," 21 September 1981, Part II, p. 9.

Newsday, (New York), Ciolli, Rita. "Blue Cross Sued Over Cancer Care," 29 September 1982, p. 6.

Newsday, (New York), Firstman, Richard C. "A Vacation With Needles," 22 April 1983, p. 7.

Newsday, (New York), Proffer, Carl R. "Becoming a Guinea Pig—to Escape Certain Death," 20 October 1983, Ideas Section, p. 5.

Newsday, (New York), "Cancer Vaccines Study," 30 March 1985.

Newsday (New York), Wingerson, Lois. "Shocking Cells into Fighting Tumors," 8 October 1985, Discovery Section, p. 11.

Newsday, (New York), Colen, B. D. "Cancer 'Cures,'" 10 December 1985, Discovery Section, p. 10.

Newsday, (New York), Hirschfeld, Neal. "Rabbi, why me?" 2 March 1986, p. 14.

Newsday, (New York), Zinman, David. "Poverty Eyed as a Factor in Cancer," 17 April 1986.

Newsday, (New York), Zinman, David. "Age and Cancer," 29 April 1986, Discovery Section, Medicine, p. 3.

Newsday, (New York), "A Double-Barreled Attack on Cancer" 27 May 1986.

Newsday, (New York), "New Test Appears to Detect All Cancers," 28 November 1986, p. 6.

Newsday, (New York), Couzens, Gerald Secor "Cancer: Fighting Back," 30 November 1986, pp. 6–7.

Newsday, (New York), "The Tradeoff In Treatment," 24 February 1987, Discovery Section, p. 3.

Newsday, (New York), Cooke, Robert. "Promising Cancer Treatment Reported," 11 June 1987, p. 4.

Newsday, (New York), "Cancer Diet," 17 June 1987, Part III, p. 1.

Newsday, (New York), Cooke, Robert. "New clues on cancer's seeds," 5 July 1988.

Newsday, (New York), "CANCER—Findings on how tumors start," 6 September 1988.

O'Neill, M. P. "Psychological aspects of cancer recovery," *Cancer,* Vol. 36, 1975, pp. 271–273.

PBS, "Currents," 28 May 1987, "Living With Cancer."

Parker, R. M.; and Hansen, Carl E. *Rehabilitation Counseling.* Boston: Allyn and Bacon, 1981.

Patterson, C. H. *Readings in Rehabilitation Counseling.* Champaign, Illinois: Stipes Publishing Co., 1960.

Perlman, Leonard G. (ed.) *The Role of Vocational Rehabilitation in the 1980's — Serving Those With Invisible Handicaps.* Washington D.C.: National Rehabilitation Association, 1978.

Pinkerton, S. S. & Nelson, S. B. "Counselor Variables Influencing Rehabilitation Outcome of Persons with Cancer," *Rehabilitation Counseling Bulletin,* 21, 1978, pp. 253–260.

Pittman, Janice L. and Mathews, Mark. "Peer Counseling: Four Exemplary Programs," *American Rehabilitation,* Vol. 10, No. 4, Oct–Nov–Dec 1984, pp. 21–24.

Potter, J. F. "Summary Statement Concerning the Successfully Treated Cancer Patient," *Cancer,* Vol. 36, No. 1, July 1975, p. 304.

Record, (New Jersey), "Cancer survival rate now as high as 41%," 15 December 1980, p. A-12.

Record, (New Jersey), "Cancer victims' odds are better than 50-50," 27 November 1984, Section A, p. 8.

Record, (New Jersey), Gorner, Peter and Lyon, Jeff. "Medicine poised for a great leap forward," 1 April 1986, Section A, p. 15.

Record, (New Jersey), "Cancer researchers insist they're not losing the war," 11 May 1986, Section A, p. 13.

Renneker, Mark and Leib, Stephen. *Understanding Cancer.* Palo Alto, California: Bull, 1979.

Rensberger, Boyce. "The Making of a Cancer Cell," *Science 84,* September 1984, pp. 28–39.

Rogers, Carl R. *Counseling and Psychotherapy.* Boston: Houghton Mifflin, 1942, p. 3, pp. 14–16.

Rogers, Carl. *Client-Centered Therapy.* Boston: Houghton Mifflin, 1951.

Rubin, S. E., Matkin, R. E., Ashley, J., Beardsley, M. M., May, V. R., Onstott, K., & Puckett, F. D. "Roles and functions of certified rehabilitation counselors," *Rehabilitation Counseling Bulletin,* 27, 1984, pp. 199–224.

Seligmann, Jean and Witherspoon, Deborah. "A New, Old Cancer Drug," *Newsweek,* June 1983.

Selikoff, I. J. and Hammond, E. C. "Cancer and the Environment," "Environmental Cancer in the Year 2000" in *Understanding Cancer,* ed. Renneker, Mark and Leib, Steven. Palo Alto, California: Bull, 1979.

Siegel, Bernie S. *Love, Medicine and Miracles.* New York: Harper and Row, 1986.

Simonton, O. Carl; Matthews-Simonton, Stephanie; and Creighton, James. *Getting Well Again.* Los Angeles, California: J. P. Tarcher, 1978.

Stolov, W. C.; and Clowers, M. R. *Handbook of Severe Disability.* Washington, D.C.: U.S. Govt. Printing Office, 1981.

Tache, Jean; Selye, Hans; and Day, Stacey B. (eds.). *Cancer, Stress and Death.* New York: Plenum, 1979.

Taylor, Celeste M. "The Rehabilitation of Persons with Cancer: Is This the Best We Can Do?," *Journal of Rehabilitation,* Oct–Nov–Dec 1984, pp. 60–62, 71.

Tyler, Leona. *The Work of the Counselor.* New York: Appleton-Century-Crofts, 1961.

U.S. Dept. of Education, National Institute of Handicapped Research, OSERS, "Psychosocial Rehabilitation of Cancer Patients," *Rehab Brief* Washington D.C.: NIHR, 14 July 1984.

U.S. Dept. of Education, O.S.E.R.S., R.S.A. "RSA 300 tabulations of characteristics of clients whose cases were closed in fy 85," Series C1 and C2, Table T012, RSA IM-87-30, 14 May 1987.

U.S. Department of Health and Human Services, Public Health Service, National Institutes of Health. *Cancer Treatment.* Medicine for the Layman Series, Lecture delivered December 13 1977 by Vincent T. DeVita, Director, National Cancer Institute, NIH Publication No. 84-1807, Washington D.C.: U.S. Government Printing Office, 1982, Reprinted February 1984.

U.S. Department of Health, Education and Welfare, Public Health Service, National Institutes of Health. *Treating Cancer.* DHEW Publication No. (NIH) 78-210, Washington D.C.: U.S. Government Printing Office, 1978.

U.S. Department of Health, Education and Welfare, Office of Human Development Services, R.S.A. Memorandum from the Commissioner Robert R. Humphreys to the RSA Regional Program Director, Seattle, Wash., March 28, 1980.

U.S. General Accounting Office Report to the Chairman, Subcommittee on Intergovernmental Relations and Human Resources, Committee on Government Operations, House of Representatives. *Cancer Patient Survival: What Progress Has Been Made?* Gaithersburg, Maryland: U.S. G.A.O., March 1987.

We Can Do!—A Unique Cancer Support Group. Descriptive brochure, Arcadia, California: 1981.

Willett, Walter C. and MacMahon, Brian. "Medical Progress, Diet and Cancer—An Overview," *New England Journal of Medicine,* Vol. 310, No. 10, 8 March 1984, pp. 633–638.

Willett, Walter C. and MacMahon, Brian. "Medical Progress, Diet and Cancer—An Overview," Second of Two Parts, *New England Journal of Medicine,* Vol. 310, No. 11, 15 March 1984, pp. 697–702.

BRITISH COLUMBIA CANCER AGENCY
LIBRARY
600 WEST 10th AVE.
VANCOUVER, B.C.   CANADA
V5Z 4E6

BRITISH COLUMBIA CANCER AGENCY
LIBRARY
600 WEST 10th AVE.
VANCOUVER, B.C.   CANADA
V5Z 4E6